Diary of a Dying AIDS Patient: Death by Betrayal

Shirl A. Jefferson

Copyright © 2024 by Shirl A. Jefferson

All rights reserved. No part of this publication may be reproduced, distributed, or transmitted in any form or by any means, including, photocopying,recording, or other electronic or mechanical methods, without the prior written permission of the copyright owner and the publisher, except in the case of brief quotations embodied in critical reviews and certain other noncommercial uses permitted by copyright law. For permission requests, write to the publisher, addressed "Attention: Permissions Coordinator," at the address below.

CITIOFBOOKS, INC.
3736 Eubank NE Suite A1
Albuquerque, NM 87111-3579
www.citiofbooks.com
Hotline: 1 (877) 389-2759
Fax: 1 (505) 930-7244

Ordering Information:
Quantity sales. Special discounts are available on quantity purchases by corporations, associations, and others. For details, contact the publisher at the address above.

Printed in the United States of America.
ISBN-13:   Paperback   979-8-89391-278-4
               eBook   979-8-89391-279-1

Library of Congress Control Number: 2024916993

Table of Contents

Chapter 1: The Growing Years 1

Chapter 2: A Fresh start 4

Chapter 3: Settled At Last 6

Chapter 4: Facing the Music 13

Chapter 5: The Date 20

Chapter 6: A New Day 25

Chapter 7: Home at Last 31

Chapter 8: Meeting the Family 38

Chapter 9: Planning a Wedding 46

Chapter 10: The Big Day at Last 56

A Mother's Tribute of Love to Her Dying Daughter 63

Diary of a Dying AIDS Patient 65

Chapter 1

The Growing Years

It was a cold and dreary November day and Kelly's spirits were low. She had been up all night studying for an economics exam and still felt that she had done poorly. Kelly was very upset because she wanted so desperately to some day become a real estate broker. It had been a dream for as long as she could remember and it seemed that the dream was slowly slipping away. She blamed her shortcomings on her boyfriend Todd.

Todd and Kelly had dated all through high school and decided to attend the same college, but ended up going separate ways. Todd was attending Harvard Law School while Kelly decided to stay close to home and was attending the University of Richmond's Robins School of Business on a full scholarship. Kelly considered herself to be a smart girl who made rational decisions except when it came to Todd. Todd had been pressuring her to have sex with him and she was just not ready. Kelly's parents were devout Christians and Kelly was their only child. They constantly doted on her and gave her everything that she wanted. She in return, always followed their rules and vowed to be the child that any parent would be proud to call their own.

How could Todd not want to respect her wishes? He had threatened to find someone who would love him and give in to his desires. While Kelly loved Todd with all her heart, she still did not want to go against the wishes of her parents and the teachings that they had instilled in her. Why did Todd want to make her life so difficult? They were many states apart and Kelly felt that Todd could still be with someone else while confessing his undying love to her. How would she know? She was faced with a dilemma that was causing her unbearable strife and sleepless nights.

Kelly finally made the long trek from class to her dorm room to wait on Todd's call. They usually talked about twice a day between classes and then again at night. Todd's phone calls helped her to make it through their time spent apart. He was the love of her life and someday they would spend their lives together as husband and wife. She got excited just thinking about their future.

When Kelly woke up, it was time for her next class. Had she slept that long, did she miss Todd's call? She began sifting through the caller ID but there was no call from him. Her mind began to race with worry. That was so out of the norm for him. Was he alright? Was he with someone else? She decided to call his cell phone in hopes for answers. The answering machine picked up on the first ring. Now she definitely became consumed with worry. Why was his phone off? She then called his dorm room, but there was no answer. What was going on? She decided to go to class and just wait for him to call her later on that evening. What a drag this class was going to be worrying about Todd and what was going on with him.

When Kelly got back to her dorm for the evening, she checked her messages and her caller ID, but still there was no call from Todd. She tried his cell phone again; still the answering machine picked up on the first ring. Kelly had had enough. She decided to call his mother to see if she had heard from Todd. Todd's mother answered the phone with a hint of sadness in her voice. "What's wrong Mrs. Thomas"; Kelly asked? You haven't heard? "Heard what'; asked Kelly? "Todd eloped this morning. He called to tell his father and me after the ceremony. He knew that we would disapprove. We wanted him to at least wait until he had finished college before making such a drastic decision. We thought that it would be you that he was going to marry. You two are so right for each other, but it seems that Brenda, the girl that he married, is pregnant and the baby is due in another seven months." All that Kelly could do was cry. Why had Todd betrayed her? He had not given her any inclination that he was even seeing someone else.

Sure they were miles apart, but she had felt that they had a strong relationship and they were able to withstand the distance. What had gone wrong? Was it because she would not give in to his advances? She had never even given any thought to any other guy. How could she have been so stupid? Was she so caught up in her dream and pleasing her parents that she hadn't noticed any differences when they talked on the phone? She hung up the phone and cried herself to sleep.

The next day, Kelly called her parents to give them the heart wrenching news and told them that she was going to take a few days off from school and come home to get her thoughts together. Her mom said that she would be waiting for her and that everything was going to be alright. They would be there to help her put the pieces together of her shattered life. God would be in control.

As time went on, Kelly eventually came to grips with losing Todd and decided that she would focus on her studies, graduating and opening her own real estate company. Kelly eventually did graduate and moved back home to South Hill, Virginia. It was a rural area and things didn't go well as originally anticipated. After five years of trying to keep a struggling business alive; she decided to move to New York City. Her parents were heart broken with her decision but told her that she had given it her all to keep her business alive and they would respect her decision.

Kelly finished up the legalities of closing her business within a month's time after making a decision to take a job with a major New York brokerage firm with her parents' blessings. She had never been so far away from them before and wondered how she would make it. She would have to make new friends, find a new church home and just basically start life over in a big city without any comforts of home.

Chapter 2

A Fresh start

When Kelly reached New York, her new employer, Mrs. Talley was waiting for her at the airport. Mrs. Talley was a middle-aged lady with salt and pepper hair and a distinguished look. Her face appeared to be friendly and she had a motherly air about her. They exchanged greetings and she told Kelly that she would take her to her to the apartment where she would be staying after they got a bite to eat. They decided on a delicatessen near La Guardia Airport.

Kelly was amazed at the diverse cultures of the persons seated in the delicatessen. They all seemed to be conversed in business and the atmosphere was not as friendly as it was at home. Mrs. Talley sensed that Kelly was uncomfortable and told her not to worry. She just needed to get used to the hustle and bustle of the city. "Besides, said Mrs. Talley, you will be so busy that you won't even be aware of what's going on around you or how lonely you are." "I know that I will be alright Mrs. Talley. Yes, I miss my parents terribly, but I am ready to immerse myself in my job."

They finally finished their meal and small talk about the brokerage business. Mrs. Talley paid the check and they left. Mrs. Talley was a stylish woman for her age. She was dressed in a Navy blue pant suit by Le Suit and strappy navy blue sandals. A scarf was donned around her neck and her hair was swept up in a bun. She was driving a black Mercedes Benz SL 550. What a classy woman, Kelly thought to herself. She hoped that she too would someday meet that statute as a broker.

They finally reached the apartment complex where the corporate members of her firm resided. She was amazed and in awe of the landscaping and the buildings. What an amazing sight to behold! Mrs. Talley informed her that Shaw's Lawncare and Landscaping was the business that was to be credited for the beautiful scenery around her. They were initially a small business located in Prince George, Virginia but had decided to take on a contract for her company. Many establishments were amazed with the landscaping of her firm and decided to give them contracts as well. Soon they were booming with business and had to expand and open a branch in the heart of New York City. I have a lot of faith in persons from small towns, so Kelly; that is one of the reasons that I decided to hire you. People from the South seem to take so much pride in their work and so that is why they are my favorites.

Kelly never dreamed that she would be living in a place like this. She always thought of New York as a big city with dirty streets and crowded pavements. Never in her wildest dreams did she think that the firm that she was going to be working for would put her up in accommodations of this sort. Mrs. Talley just smiled at Kelly's astonishment and patted her on the back. "Are you ready to see where you will be staying?" Kelly said that she was, and Mrs. Talley entered the security code on the gate's key pad and they went through.

Mrs. Talley stayed for about thirty minutes to help Kelly get settled and told her that a car would be arriving at 8:00 AM the following morning to take her to the office. After Mrs. Talley left, Kelly settled down and called her parents. They were eager to hear her voice and had lots of questions to ask her. She informed them that she was tired but would call them on tomorrow to fill them in on all of the details of her new home and her job.

Chapter 3

Settled At Last

Kelly was awake before her alarm clock went off. She felt refreshed and vibrant. For her first day on her new job; she selected a classic black suit designed by Donna Karen. Her shoes were black stilettos made by Nine West and her accessories were silver. Kelly completed her look with a black handbag by Coach. Her make up was done carefully so as not to look as if she was artificial and her hair was impeccable.

She would miss her stylist from home, Pat. Pat was the owner of Turnin' Headz in Petersburg, Virginia and was a master weaver who always did an outstanding job with Kelly's hair. Pat was Todd's cousin and she and Kelly had quickly become good friends when she first met Todd. Her new stylist was a girl recommended by her best friend Karen. Karen had grown up in New York but had often spent her summers in Virginia with her grandmother. She and Karen had always been very close and shared their innermost secrets with one another and had the same ambitious outlook on life; so she trusted Karen's choice of stylist and could not wait to meet her. Karen's hair was always the bomb and Kelly had faith that Cindy would work the same type of miracle on her hair as Pat had done because she would not have the time to go to Virginia every week to have her hair done.

After getting ready for work, Kelly sat in her breakfast nook starring out at the beautiful landscaping. What a view; if only she could share it with Todd. The loudspeaker blaring with the voice of the security guard startled her. "Ms. Russell, your driver is here." "Okay, thanks, I will be right down". Kelly swiftly gathered up her things and headed downstairs. She was greeted by a limo driver who was caramel in color, long, well-cared for dreads and a body that said he was an avid lover of somebody's gym. He definitely looked the part of a ladies man. His name was Bennie and what a handsome specimen he was; but she was not ready to get on the dating scene yet. Todd was still a force to be reckoned with but she knew that she would have to forget about him. He was married with a child on the way. Why did she bother to even wait for him all those years?

Kelly made small talk with the driver on the way to the office. She found out that he had played in the NFL as a quarterback for the Philadelphia Eagles and had sustained injuries that cost him his career and his family. He and a few of his team mates had gone out to celebrate a victorious win against the Washington Redskins. He had a little too much to drink but decided that he was still okay to drive. His wife insisted that he allow her to drive but he assured her that he was okay. As they attempted to get onto the freeway, he over negotiated his turn onto the ramp and ended up in the pathway of a tractor trailer. All that he could remember of the accident was the sound of screeching metal and the eerie screams from his wife. The next day, he awoke from a coma with his mother and his preacher by his bedside. They gave him the chilling news that his wife and unborn child did not survive the crash. Bennie had sustained major injuries to his right leg that caused him to limp when he walked and sometimes gave out on him. After recovering from his injuries, he was informed that he would no longer be able to play football. Bennie had met Mrs. Talley years ago when she first opened her brokerage firm and decided to see if she had any positions open as a limo driver. She did, and he accepted the position graciously. Since the death of his wife and unborn son, Bennie vowed that he would never drink alcohol again. He loved his wife very much and even though it had been five years since her death, he was not yet ready to release his heart to another woman. In his off time he often went to the gym as a way to release stress and to exercise his legs. When he was not in the gym, he played his saxophone for mental therapy. Finally they reached her office and he got out to open her door. She bid him a good day and promised him that they would continue their conversation when he came back to pick her up that evening.

Kelly got on the elevator and was eager to start her new job. She was humming "Oh Happy Day" as she walked past the receptionist. Mrs. Talley was there to greet Kelly at her office and introduced her to her executive secretary. She had a small build and looked like a plain Jane with a smile that was infectious. Kelly knew that she would like Janet working for her. Janet took Kelly's briefcase out of her hand and directed her to the conference room on the third floor. There she was greeted by a man with such a warm smile. He was the CEO of training and his name was Mr. Seward. Mr. Seward appeared to be a man of distinction and had a hint of a swagger. He was well dressed and she knew that all of the women in the firm were competing for his attention. She knew that she would definitely have to stay focused on her job because his smile was so warm and inviting and his eyes were a soft hue of brown that seemed to sparkle. In some ways he resembled Todd and she did not want any reminders of him. Her life with him was over and she swore that she would settle into her new job and forget all about him.

During the orientation; all of the new hires took turns introducing themselves and what department they would be working in. They all seemed to have come from diverse backgrounds with extensive knowledge of the brokering business. She knew that she would like working for this firm and looked forward to personally meeting all of her co-workers.

Orientation was an all day event and Kelly was glad when it was finally over. She went downstairs to the lobby to wait for her driver. She did not have to wait long. Once she stepped off of the elevator, Bennie was there and took her briefcase from her. She remembered the conversation from this morning and was eagerly waiting to learn more about him. He was such a down to earth person and had a personality that reminded her of someone from the South. Benny asked Kelly if she wanted to join him for dinner. She said that she had nothing else to do and enjoyed his company. Benny told her that he knew of a nice restaurant not far from her office that served southern cuisine. She admitted that it sounded good because she did not know when the last time was that she had eaten a good home cooked meal. Benny was right; the menu was filled with mouth watering foods and desserts. She had a hard time deciding what she wanted to eat so she allowed Benny to choose for her. He recommended that she try the fried catfish, collard greens and macaroni and cheese. The meal was scrumptious and they decided to top it off with homemade apple pie and a bowl of vanilla ice cream. Kelly enjoyed hearing about Benny's childhood and his life in the NFL. It was hard for her to believe that some woman had not scooped him up. He was quite a catch! Benny was from South Carolina and had received a full scholarship to Howard University. Scouts from the Washington Redskins, Atlanta Falcons and Carolina Panthers were watching him from his first year at Howard. He decided to go with the Redskins because he and his wife had met while at Howard University and she wanted to stay near her ailing parents. After the accident, Bennie felt as though he was obligated to take care of them since he was the cause of their daughter not being there to care for her parents. He missed his family and friends in South Carolina but this was his way of giving back for the time that he had taken their daughter away from them. He said that he usually went home at least twice a year. One of his friends in the NFL's mom had a home health care business and provided respite care for his in-laws. Benny was an only child but had two half sisters whom he adored. They all still resided in South Carolina and had children and busy lives. They would attempt to visit him at least once a year. He enjoyed their time together and wished that he could see them more often. They had always been a close knit family and enjoyed the time that they spent together. Well, that was water under the bridge and he could not undue the loss that he had caused his in-laws. Finally, they reached her building and Benny got out to open her door. They said their good byes and she headed into her building. Once she got in the house, she sat down to call her parents. Her mom answered the phone eager to hear how her first day went. Kelly informed her mother that she had met her executive ecretary and the other brokers that would be working with her. She said that they had not done much of anything because orientation had lasted all day. She said that she felt that she was going to like the job and the people that she worked with. They talked for about thirty more minutes and Kelly told her mom that it had been a long day and she needed to get ready for bed.

After taking a long bubble bath, Kelly fixed herself a cup of tea and sat down to read her Bible. She could not figure out why some woman had not yet snatched up Bennie. He was quite a catch who appeared to have his priorities in order and was a believer of God as well. Kelly felt that he and her secretary, Janet would be a great match. She would arrange for them to somehow cross each other's path. Her mother had warned her years ago that match making was not a good thing. If things did not work out, then she would have to face the possibility that they could be upset with her and a friendship would be lost. Kelly was certain that this would not be the case for Bennie and Janet. They both had nice personalities, believed in God and were steadfast in their devotion to the higher power. Most of all, they both needed companionship. While she couldn't believe that she was passing up one heck of a hunk; she was just not ready to jump in a relationship and just wanted to focus on her new job, learn the city, get to know herself a little bit better and what destination her life was going to take.

Finally, her first week of work was over. Kelly decided that after putting in over sixty hours in her first week; she was definitely in need of pampering. Kelly got up early on Saturday morning and called Ms. Talley to see where she could go for a spa day. Ms. Talley told Kelly that she patronized a spa not far from her building. It was owned by a lady named Nita. Nita had been in the city for about five years and built her clientele up nicely. People loved to go there because the atmosphere was always warm and inviting and she was also good at what she did. Her mom would sometimes stop by with homemade meals that were to die for. Ms. Talley told Kelly that she would go with her if she didn't mind the company. "Sure" said Kelly. "Should I phone Bennie?" "No" said Ms. Talley. I will swing by and get you. That way, we won't have to hold him up all day. Besides, let's make a girl's day out and hit the malls and catch a movie later on." "That sounds like a winner to me", said Kelly. I will be ready in about an hour. I will see you then".

Ms. Talley was right. The spa was decorated with scenes of tranquility and painted in soft pastel hues. It was an amazing place and she was certain that she would enjoy her time there. She was introduced to Kevin. He would be the person giving her a pedicure and manicure and his wife Jennifer would do her facial and massage. The service that she received was great and she was sure that she would make it a weekly visit.

After their visit to the spa, Ms. Talley and Kelly headed to Nita's to get their hair done and then headed to the Mall. Coming from a small rural area, Kelly could not believe the size of the mall. It was spacious. It had eight floors with over 300 stores! How in the world could anyone possibly know where to even start to shop? Ms. Talley told her that the floors were divided according to merchandise. For example, furniture was on the first two floors, salons and spas were on the third floor, casual clothing and sportswear on the fourth floor and dress clothes on the fifth floor. All departments were color coded on a map strategically placed on all floors, so if she forgot what floor she needed to go to; all she had to do was go to the map. Kelly and Ms. Talley spent over three hours in the mall before finally going to the eighth floor to catch a movie. Kelly was too tired to eat and told Ms. Talley that she just wanted to go home and crash. Ms. Talley told her that was fine because she was kinda tired too. Ms. Talley told Kelly that she would be by around 8:00 the next morning to pick her up for church.

The next day, the church service was awesome. Ms. Talley was a member of Pleasant Grove Baptist Church and the pastor, Rev. Gooding was truly a man of God. His sermon, "Ima do Me, You do You" was so moving and she knew that this was the church that she would join. When the invitation was extended, Kelly quickly rose to go to the front of the church. She was greeted by Deacon Davis and escorted to the fellowship hall by the church clerk, Mrs. Draughan. When the reached the fellowship hall for the clerk to take her information; a lady was passing through to take some children to the restroom. Mrs. Draughan told Kelly that the lady passing through was the pastor's wife. Her name was Marlene. Ms. Draughan introduced them once Marlene came out of the restroom. Kelly couldn't help but notice the bracelet that Marlene was wearing. It had the greek lettering that said she was a member of Delta Sigma Theta Sorority, Inc. Kelly told Marlene that she too was a Delta and was new to the area and had been looking for a chapter to join. Marlene told Kelly that she would give her the location of her chapter and meeting dates and time after church. Kelly thanked her and left to join Mrs. Draughan in the sanctuary. After church, they decided to go to Shoney's for breakfast because they could get the buffet and not have to wait as long as some of the other restaurants. Shoney's was nice and reminded Kelly of home. She then thought about how much she missed her parents. She definitely had to find a weekend out of her busy schedule to go and visit with them. She had been putting it off because she did not want to run into Todd and his wife. She was not yet over him and did not know whether or not she could handle it. Her mother and some of the elders in her home church had vowed that God had allowed her to persevere when faced with adversity in the past and He would sure get her through this. Why did she doubt what God could do? This was definitely one of those times that she questioned her faith. How would she react if she saw them? Could she speak and not get emotional? One thing was for sure; she could no longer put off seeing her parents just because she did not want to face Todd or relive the events of the day that she found out about his infidelities. God was in charge and would get her through this difficult time. She knew that this was true because He had brought her out of so many other circumstances in the past. She also remembered her mother telling her that some people are in your life for a season and some for a life time. If Todd could not respect her feelings about wanting to wait until marriage before they engage in sexual acts; then he certainly was not the man for her. It was best that she found out who he was before she gave herself to him completely.

Chapter 4

Facing the Music

Well, Friday had finally arrived and Kelly was beat after the sixty hours that she had put in for the week. She wanted to just spend a quiet and uneventful weekend at home lounging around and catching up on her reading. She had just purchased five hundred dollars worth of books last week to fill those long boring fall evenings that were quickly approaching. She had phoned her mother earlier in the week to let her know that she would be coming home for a visit this weekend and knew that she had better stick to the plan because she knew that her parents were eager to see her and to hear more about her life in the "Big Apple". She was not going to let them down because she knew that her mom had already started preparing an elegant meal and her father had probably taken the liberty of purchasing fresh flowers of whatever was in bloom for the season. Kelly had always loved flowers and her father always adorned the house with flowers of every fragrant and bloom whenever Kelly had shown signs of disappointment or just plan sad. Her father always knew how to cheer up his "baby girl".

When her alarm clock went off at 5:00 a.m. on Saturday morning, Kelly hit the snooze button and pulled the covers over her head. How she wished that she could sleep just a little bit longer but she wanted to get on the highway by 6:00 a.m. in order to beat the weekend traffic. She finally decided to get up about fifteen minutes later. After saying a quick prayer, hitting the shower and pouring herself a mug of coffee; Kelly felt like she was prepared to face anything. After checking the fuel levels in her car, Kelly was ready to hit the road. She put a CD by BeeBee and CeCe Winans in the CD player, set her car on cruise control and jumped on the freeway. It was smooth sailing until she reached Maryland. Kelly decided to stop at the Maryland House to freshen up and get something to eat. She also needed to stretch her legs because she had driven for almost an hour and a half with bumper to bumper traffic.

Once Kelly had finished eating, she decided to call her mom to let her know that she would be pulling up to their house in about three hours. The traffic in Maryland had been horrendous once she reached Maryland. I should be pulling into their driveway around 4:00 p.m. Kelly told her mom that she had stopped to get a bite to eat but still had room for her home cooked meal.

Kelly reached her parents' house around 5:00 p.m. She grabbed her suitcase from the trunk and ran through her parents' house letting them know that she was home. Her mother yelled for her to come out to the back deck. When Kelly reached the deck; it was full. Her mom had neglected to tell her that they were planning a cook out in her honor. She had just wanted to spend a quiet evening with her parents and get on the highway after church. Was she ready to face her old friends and not have to explain the situation between her and Todd. They had a small knit community and everybody knew everything about everybody. She could not be mad at her parents and would just have to face whatever questions or comments that people had.

The crowd of people at her parents' house quickly grew and they had ran out of buns and ice. Kelly's mom asked her if she would go to the local supermarket. Kelly was hesitant at first but decided to go anyway. When she reached the parking lot, she saw Todd and his wife get out of a car near hers. What would she say? Could she just pretend not to see them? Todd's wife did not know who she was but she was sure that Todd had told her. They had a lot of history and she was still friends with his family. They were all excited when Kelly and Todd had been a couple and always felt that they would someday get married. With a fake smile plastered on her face, Kelly finally exited the car and spoke to Todd and his wife. Todd introduced his wife to Kelly and Kelly extended her hand to greet her. They all entered the store and went their separate ways. This was an awkward situation for Kelly. She hoped that Todd's wife did not notice the whimsical look on her face. Why did Todd have to still look so good? He could still make heart beat with excitement. Kelly felt tears start to well in her eyes and she quickly went to the ladies room before anyone could see her. She threw water on her face and patted her face and eyes dry. Kelly regained her composure and left out to get the items that her mother wanted her to get. When she reached the checkout, Todd and his wife were checking out too. She told them that she was in a hurry to get the items that her mother had sent her to get and maybe next time, she would be able to chat with them and turned to leave. What a scar Todd had left on her heart but she knew that eventually she would heal; but just how long would that take?

When Kelly arrived back at her parents' house, her best friend Money had arrived. Money and Kelly had been friends every since first grade. When they got to the high school, they both joined the ROTC. Kelly hated it but Money decided to join the military upon graduation and Kelly went off to college. They had not seen each other in about seven or eight years but stayed in touch by phone calls and face book. Money had just returned from her third tour of the Iraq/Afghanistan wars. This was certainly a surprise that Kelly's mother had kept secret. After giving her mother the items from the grocer, Kelly and Money moved to the side of the deck and conversed about old times. She told Money how she had ran into Todd and his new wife and how awkward it was meeting them for the first time as a couple. She admitted that it was hard on her seeing them together and how she had broke out in tears and had to go to the restroom to regain her composure. She had often wondered how it would be if she ever saw them together. Would she be angry with Todd because of his betrayal or would say just give it over to God and move on? She decided on the latter. Kelly and Money talked for hours even after the other guests had gone home. Kelly finally looked at her watch and saw that it was going on midnight. She told Money that she had better head in because she promised her parents that she was going with them to church before leaving to go home. Money told her that it was good to see her and that she would drive to New York to pay her a visit. She had ten days of leave left and would come up on Friday and leave on Sunday. Kelly told her that was fine and she was looking forward to spending time together. Money told her that she was not sure if she was going to make it to church because she had just returned from the Middle East and had not yet gotten acclimated to the time change but she would try.

When Kelly entered the doors of her home church, Gethsemane; she saw that Money was indeed there and some of her other friends from high school. It was good to be on familiar territory and she could feel the warmth and love from all of the people that she had grown up with. The pastor told her that it was good to see her again and informed the congregation about her job as a real estate agent in a brokerage firm on Wall Street. He went on to tell her how proud that she had made her folks from back home and he hoped that she would be able to join them again soon.

After the service, Kelly went up to give her pastor and his wife a hug and told them that she missed them terribly but had found a church that she enjoyed. She told them how impressive Rev. Gooding was at her first time at his church. He was definitely a man of God and preached God's word with conviction. What she liked most of all was the way that he showed love to his wife and children. They were definitely a match made in heaven and she was sure God had an abundance of blessings in store for him. She went on to say that she had the opportunity to meet some of the other church members and thought that she was going to like this church and was looking forward to working with the Missionary Ministry. After speaking with him for about ten minutes, she bid him fair well and joined up with her mother and Money who were waiting for her. Her mother told her that her father was waiting for them at Denny's and that they should hurry if she planned on getting on the highway at a reasonable time.

They left the restaurant about 1:00 and Kelly told her mom that she was going to pack and get on the road in about another hour which would put her home at about 10:00 or 11:00 p.m. She would take a half day off from work so that she could get some rest before going in. Being a real estate agent on Wall Street was a lucrative but competitive market and she had to work long hours just to stay on top. Kelly and her parents sat out on the deck for about forty minutes just catching up on what was going on in their lives since they had not gotten the opportunity to talk that much since her arrival. It was good to be home but now she must head back to face the hustle and bustle of city life.

It was about 11:30 when Kelly pulled into her garage. She quickly phoned her parents to let them know that she had arrived home safely and was going to take a long hot bath and hit the bed. Kelly called the messaging center to let them know that she would not be in until about noon tomorrow. She set her alarm for 10:00 a.m. and got into bed. Kelly did not realize how tired she was until the next morning. It felt like every part of her body had been beaten. She sighed and got up anyway. Kelly decided that the trip had taken a toll on her and she would only work for a few hours. At about 11:15 a.m, Bennie was buzzing her penthouse to see if she was ready. She assured him that she was and would be down in a few minutes. She just needed to put the finishing touches on her make-up and grab her brief case. He told her that he would be waiting for her in the lobby. Bennie was such a gentleman that he always took her brief case for her. He really did need a special woman in his life and she smiled to herself and vowed that she would arrange a chance meeting soon.

When Kelly arrived to work, Ms. Talley was in the hallway and asked her if she enjoyed her weekend. She said that she did and it was a much needed trip. Kelly then went to Janet's office to retrieve whatever messages she had. After talking with Janet for a while, she asked her what her plans were for the upcoming weekend. Janet said that she had no plans and wanted to know why. I just have someone that I want you to meet. I will tell you more about it later on in the week.

Kelly decided to call it quits about 6:00 p.m. and called Bennie to let him know that she was ready to leave for the evening. He told her that he would be downstairs in another ten minutes. She told him that was fine and she would meet him in the lobby. When Kelly got in the car, Bennie asked her if she would like to join him for dinner before going home because he wanted to know how her weekend went and if she had run into Todd and his wife. She agreed to have dinner with him and had grown accustomed to sharing her dinner meal with him. She had immersed herself in her work and had not taken the opportunity to meet a lot of people. Most of her acquaintances had been people that she worked with and only shared a casual working relationship. This evening, they decided to have dinner at an outdoors bistro. The food was just delectable and Kelly really enjoyed Bennie's choice in restaurants. He was quite the food connoisseur.

Bennie told Kelly that he wanted to hear about her weekend at home and not to leave out any juicy details. Kelly laughed and told him that he was worse than a gossiping woman. She told him how her parents had put together a surprise cook out for her and invited all of her friends. Her best friend was also there. She was returning from the Middle East and was on leave before returning to her next duty station. "As a matter of fact, she will be here this weekend", said Kelly. "You will like her. We have been friends since elementary school. We took ROTC together in high school. Money liked the military life and joined after graduating from high school and I chose college with a professional career. I could not have made it in the military." When Kelly started telling Bennie how she had run into Todd and his new wife in the market; he noticed that tears started to well in her eyes. Bennie dried her tears and told her that it was okay and he would not pressure her to tell him anymore. He changed the subject and told her that he had been out of town the weekend himself. He had gone to see his wife's parents to make sure that they had enough food and that their bills were taken care of. Their care giver would usually call him once the food got low or a bill was due. The care givers didn't have to call him too often because whenever he visited them; he always left extra money just in case an emergency arose. They talked a little bit more about his in-laws until Kelly asked him if he would like to meet a friend of hers. He initially said that he did not know if he was ready to meet someone yet. A lot of women might not understand the relationship that he had with his in-laws and he would always be there for them as long as they needed him. Kelly assured him that Janet was a nice Christian lady and the meeting would be strictly platonic. After a lot of pleading, Bennie finally agreed to meet Janet on Friday evening after work. They would all go to get something to eat and catch a movie. Kelly was so elated that she grabbed Bennie by the cheeks and planted a huge kiss on his forehead. Kelly was so happy that Bennie had finally agreed to see someone that she prayed extra hard that night to thank God for answering her prayers and sending a soul mate for her dear friend Bennie. She knew that even though she was attracted to Bennie at their first meeting, they could never be more than friends. His job as her friend and confidant was all that he could ever be for her and she was glad that he had been there for her on all those difficult and trying days. With him as a friend, she didn't think about Todd as much as she had before. Sure it hurt her to see the man that she thought she would spend the rest of her life with married to someone else. This weekend was evident that she needed to stop indulging herself into her job and live again. Besides, she needed to give Bennie the time that he needed to develop a relationship with Janet.

When Kelly got to work the next day, she told Janet all about Bennie. At first Janet was hesitant but agreed to go only because Kelly would be going along with them. It was then settled. They would leave work promptly at 5:00 and get a bite to eat wherever Bennie decided they would go and then check out the movie, Dances with Wolves. They were going to catch the 7:00 show so it would give enough time for Bennie and Janet to get acquainted. Kelly was not going to tell her mom that she had been playing match maker.

When Bennie arrived to pick Kelly up that afternoon, he noticed that she was more bubbly than usual and he wanted to know why. Kelly told him that Janet had also agreed to the date on Friday. She babbled on and on about Janet to Bennie. She knew that she had to assist Janet in purchasing a new wardrobe because Bennie always looked so debonair in his street clothes, hell; he looked good in his uniform. She decided that she would invite Janet to lunch with her one day during the week and take her on a shopping spree at her expense. She did not want to hurt Janet's feelings about her style of dress, so she was just going to tell her that she wanted to buy her a few outfits as a thank you for the work that she had been doing for her, but most importantly; just for being a good friend that she greatly treasured.

Chapter 5

The Date

Kelly woke up on Friday morning before her alarm went off. She took her time tidying up her place before getting in the shower. She had so much time to spare, that she was in the lobby talking to the security guard when Bennie came to pick her up. "Why are you looking so eager to go to work this morning?" Kelly quickly reminded him what day it was and could not wait for the work day to be over. When she got in her building, she quickly ran to Janet's office to make sure that she had not changed her mind about going out after work. Janet was a very shy and reserved person and Kelly thought that she would change her mind. Kelly noticed that Janet was wearing one of the outfits that she had selected for her. It looked nice on her. Kelly decided that would convince Janet to allow her to pin her hair in an up do before they left the office so that she wouldn't look too conservative.

Truly Bennie had done his homework as usual. He had selected a quaint little restaurant with just enough lighting that made for a romantic atmosphere. A jazz group was performing for their entertainment. What an enchanted evening! Kelly had to quickly strike up a conversation because her mind was drifting back to Todd again. Why had she allowed him to have such an impact on her life? She vowed that after tonight, would definitely devise a strategy to get her mind off of Todd.

The waiter finally arrived to take their orders. Bennie ordered a bottle of Moscato to go along with their meal. Moscato is a Brazilian wine and it went perfectly with their meal of xinxim de galinha, a dish made of chicken cooked with lime, garlic, ginger, coconut milk and crushed cashews. It is fried with a vegetable oil. When their food had arrived, Kelly could not wait to indulge in it. She teased Bennie that he must have been saving this place for a special day. He said that he and some of his team mates would sometimes eat there whenever they played the Giants. He knew that they would like it and besides; it was walking distance from the Cinema. They all engaged in small talk and Kelly was surprised at how comfortable Janet appeared to be while talking to Bennie. It seemed that they had an immediate chemistry and had a lot in common as well. Kelly could not believe that Janet was such an avid football fan and she guessed that was one of the reasons why Janet was comfortable talking to Bennie. She was glad that they were getting along and patted herself on the back.

After they had finished their meal, Bennie suggested that they try a Brazilian banana cake for dessert. The girls did not want any dessert and thought they just wanted to enjoy the conversation and music until it was time for them to go to the movies. The group was performing a rendition by of "I Don't Have the Heart" by James Ingram. Bennie asked Janet if she would like to dance. She obliged and when they stepped on the floor, it seemed as though they were having an intimate moment and she was glad that everything was going so smoothly for them. Just as she took her eyes off of them; someone patted her on the shoulder and asked her if she wanted to dance. She didn't really want to, but did not want to come off as a square, so she said yes. After all, it couldn't be that bad and he was a nice looking guy. Once they got on the floor, he informed her that he they worked in the same building and that he had noticed her when she first came to the firm. He told her that his name was Kevin and he was an investment banker. He was an alumnus of Georgetown University and had majored in Public Policy. He came from a large family of five brothers and two sisters. His father divorced his mother when he was in middle school and he immersed himself in his studies to ease the pain of losing his father. He had not seen him since the divorce. His mother worked three jobs to meet the needs of the family along with assistance from his grandparents. He did well in school and had received a full scholarship to Georgetown University. He attended Syracuse University for grad school and had landed an internship on Wall Street. He had done well and they had offered him a full time position in the department that he was currently working for. After the dance, Kelly thanked him and headed back to their table. He followed her and asked her what her plans were for later on in the evening. She told him that she and her friends were leaving in a few minutes to see Tyler Perry's new movie. He told her that he had nothing else to do and if she would mind him joining them. He was supposed to meet a friend for drinks but had gotten stood up. Kelly told him that she did not mind and besides, she was not in the mood to be a third wheel. When Bennie and Janet got back to the table, she asked them if they were okay with Kevin going with them to the movies. They told her that they had no objection and it was nice to have someone tag along to keep Kelly company so that he and Janet could get better acquainted, so they decided to make it a double date.

The movie left the girls teary eyed and they decided that they needed to go to the ladies' room and freshen up their make-up. When they came out, the guys were waiting for them and eager to hear what they had to say about the movie. They all agreed that it was sad but that's just how life turns out sometimes. The good people always seem to suffer and be hurt by those that they trust the most. Sometimes you think that you know a person, but you really don't.

It was getting late and Kelly decided that she wanted to turn in for the evening. The others agreed that it had been an eventful day and they were all a bit tired and wanted to just crash. Kelly and Kevin exchanged cell phone numbers and agreed to stay in touch.

When Kelly got home, she phoned her mom to tell her all about her activities of the day and how much fun she had. She also told her that she had met an exciting guy who worked at the same firm that she did and could not wait to get better acquainted with him. They talked for a little while longer and finally Kelly told her mom that she needed to get off the phone and get some rest because Money was coming to visit her this weekend. Kelly knew that she needed to be refreshed whenever she and Money got together because they always had an eventful time with lots of ground to cover. Money was a free spirit and loved to party. She felt that the sky was the limit and the world had a lot to offer.

Kelly got up early Saturday morning to pick up a few things to make Money's weekend great. Her first stop was to the market to pick up all of Money's favorite food. She picked up some wine as well but knew that she would have to go to the package store because Money loved Hennessey. After that, Kelly went to bath and body works to get pick up some things to make a welcome basket to place in the guest room for Money.

By the time that Kelly arrived home, she had just enough time to put away all of the things that she had purchased before she had to pick Money up from the airport. Money's flight was scheduled to be on time and Kelly had to hurry to get there on time.

When Kelly arrived at the airport, she could not find a parking spot and had to circle the parking lot three times. "What a mess," she exclaimed. Kelly walked briskly to the gate where Money's flight was to disembark. By the time that she pushed her way through the crowd, Money was already walking towards her. They ran to each other and embraced for a moment. Kelly then placed Money's luggage on a cart and headed to where she was parked. Once they reached the car, Kelly told Money that she had already picked up her favorite drink and all of her favorite foods. She was in for a real treat as far as the meal that she was going to prepare for her. Kelly was a country girl and her mom had taught her how to cook before she was a teenager. Mature women in the south always believed that the way to get a husband was to be a good cook, among other things.

After Kelly had prepared the food, she went out on the patio to join Money, who had already started to indulge in the Hennessey. Money told Kelly that she was tired of the military and was planning to retire. She said that she was getting too old to take orders from people and that her body could no longer take the physical strains that it once had. Money told Kelly that she was planning to move back to Texas with her family. She would return to visit her sometimes but was going to spend her retirement years exploring exotic places. She felt that she had no real connections to Virginia now that her youngest son had graduated and had moved to Florida. Money had a bitter divorce and vowed that she would not totally give her heart to another man. She would never again be in a committed relationship, besides; she was having too much fun.

The food was finally done and Money and Kelly were starving. Money told Kelly that she had not eaten such a scrumptious meal in a long time but Kelly needed to know that while the food was good; she could never top her in the kitchen! The two agreed to a square off at a later date. Kelly told Money that she had been cooking every since she was knee high to a duck and she would teach her not to go up against her until she had taken some lessons in the kitchen.

Money and Kelly spent the rest of the evening just reminiscing about old times and the plans that they had for their futures. Kelly told Money that she was had not given much thought to a relationship in her future. Todd had hurt her immensely and she was afraid to trust again. She said that she did want to get married someday and give her parents lots of grandbabies because it sucked to be an only child. Kelly went on to tell Money that she did meet a nice guy that worked in her building and that they had gone to the movies and dancing later. He seemed okay but she would need more time to feel him out.

The next morning, Kelly got up to fix breakfast for herself and Money and then started to get ready for church. She knocked on the spare bedroom door to see if Money was going to join her. Money told Kelly that she did not feel like getting up and would see her when she got back. When Kelly returned three hours later, Money was up and packing for her flight back home. When they reached the airport, they said their teary goodbyes and Kelly headed back to her car. She hated the thought of her friend moving so far away from her. Oh well, she would just have to face the fact that people were going to enter and exit her life as long as she lived on this earth. She had developed a strong faith and knew that God would not put any more on her than she could bear. It was certainly God who had gotten her over her terrible breakup with Todd.

Chapter 6

A New Day

When Kelly got to work on Monday morning, a crystal vase of red roses with white carnations greeted her. How beautiful she thought but could not think of why she was so deserving of such a lovely gift. The card read, "Thanks for a great evening and would like to have lunch with you today." Kelly was stunned and did not know what to make of such a gorgeous gift. She scanned the directory until she found Kevin's extension and dialed his number. He had such a sensual voice and Kelly had goose bumps forming just at the sound of his voice. "I take it that you saw the roses." "Yes, replied Kelly, and they are just too much." "Anything for such a lovely lady," said Kevin. Kevin told Kelly that he was happy that he had ran into them on Friday night and that it was one of the most enjoyable times that he had seen in a long time and would like to share more times like that with her in the future. Kelly agreed and informed him that she needed to hang up and prepare for an important conference call but would meet him for lunch at the bistro across from their office building. Kelly could not wait to get back to her office to call her mom and tell her about Kevin. She knew that her mom would be happy for her decision to start dating again.

When Bennie met Kelly in the lobby that afternoon, she was grinning from ear to ear and had such a warm glow on her face. He asked her why she was looking so radiant after having worked all day in such a stress filled position. Kelly told him about the roses that she had received from Kevin and that they had went out for lunch together and how he had wanted to spend more time with her. She agreed that she was smitten with him but was still unsure if she wanted to develop a serious relationship just yet. Bennie told her that he enjoyed spending time with Janet and that she reminded him so much of his late wife. He said that a Godly woman was such a rare commodity in New York. They went to church together on Sunday and out to brunch later. He had spent some time with his wife's parents on Saturday evening and had prepared their dinner for them to have on Sunday. The nurse aide informed him that they were doing well but did not want to go out too much these days. He said that he would love to spend more time with Janet and get to know her a little bit more.

The summer finally came to an end and the days seemed long and uneventful. Kelly enjoyed the spring and summer seasons because fall and winter seemed so dreary since her break up with Todd. She was thankful that things were getting much easier for her and that she had a lot to be thankful for. She had a new and fulfilling job and new friends. She and Kevin were dating each other exclusively and things could not have been better, so why was she feeling so blue?

Kelly was snapped back to the present by the blaring of the phone. Who could be calling her so early on a Saturday morning? Kelly looked at the caller ID and saw that it was Janet. Janet was calling to tell her that Bennie had invited her to go with him to visit his in-laws. She was kind of nervous about going and wanted some advice from Kelly. "Girl, don't sweat the small stuff." I am sure that things will be okay. Bennie is such a great guy and he would not have asked you to go if he thought that it was a problem. I am sure that he has talked it over with them and they gave him the okay. He has a great relationship with his in-laws and besides; what do you have to lose?" They talked a little bit longer and Janet said that she would call Bennie and tell him that she was going. She asked Kelly what her plans were for the day and she said that she was going to go shopping for some things to redecorate her house for the fall and just have a lazy day. She wanted to get it done because she was going to visit with her parents next weekend for their 50th wedding anniversary. Her aunt was planning a surprise dinner for them and she was going to take them out for a while so that her aunt could get everything prepared. Janet told Kelly that she would call her when she returned on Sunday or talk with her at work on Monday.

At 7:30 on Monday morning, Kelly's phone rang. Ms. Talley was on the other end and had a somber voice. "What's wrong Ms. Talley", Kelly asked? I just called to let you know that I will be picking you up for work this morning because Bennie is not back yet. His mother-in-law took ill over the weekend and he is staying longer than he anticipated. Janet is going to stay with him and I have already phoned a temp agency to get you a secretary. They will be sending someone around ten this morning. Kelly thanked Ms. Talley and told her that she would be ready when she arrived. After hanging up with Ms. Talley, Kelly called Bennie's cell to check on him and Janet. Kelly told him that Ms. Talley had called and gave her the message about his mother-in-law. "Why didn't you call me, Bennie?" Bennie told her that everything had happened so fast and that he figured Ms. Talley would let her know. "So how is she," Kelly asked? "She's doing as well as can be expected. She fell and broke her hip while trying to get out of bed to get a drink of water. She's diabetic and gets thirsty a lot. The nurse usually leaves a pitcher of water on her night stand. There was a replacement nurse this weekend and I guess she forgot to leave some water on the nightstand. The doctors performed surgery on her last night and said that it would be touch and go for the next seventy-two hours because of her age. As long as she does not get an infection; everything should heal nicely. I will probably be here until she goes home. Once she gets out of the hospital; she will need to go to rehab for a couple of weeks. I will be bringing Janet back some time today, so you will only have to put up with a temp for today and Ms. Talley will get one of the interns from the office to chauffer you until I return. I hope that it won't be but a couple of weeks." "Well, take care and let me know if there is something that I can do. I can come the weekend and prepare some meals for you guys. You know that I can throw down in the kitchen said Kelly." "I will definitely hold you to that and I will be in touch later on in the week and you have a great day."

By the time that Kelly got off the phone with Bennie, Ms. Talley was there to take her to the office. Ms. Talley told Kelly that she would get to meet Bennie's replacement some time during the day. If all went well, Kelly would have her friend Bennie back in a couple of weeks and

Janet would be taking the day off. Bennie would be driving her back some time later today, so she would have a temp executive assistant for just today unless Janet needed another to rest. Janet was a dedicated employee and Ms. Talley did not anticipate her missing any more time unless it was absolutely necessary.

When Kelly reached her office, Mr. Seward was waiting for her in the receptionist area. "To what do I owe this pleasure," asked Kelly. "I just wanted to let you know that I have interviewed your assistant for the day and thought that I would personally come here to give you a brief description of what to expect. She's highly qualified and works for a temp agency because of the flexibility. Her name is Dee.

She was was wounded while serving in Iraq and receives extensive treatment at the VA hospital. Her MOS while serving in the military was a Human Resource Specialist. She was injured while a bomb exploded at the Post Exchange. She had gone there to get office supplies because supplies could not get to their base because the bridges had been blown up. A military police had saved her life. He threw her to the ground and laid on her when the bomb exploded. He was killed and she survived but lost one of her feet. The accident left her damaged psychologically as well but she needed to do something to keep her mind in tact. You will like her Kelly. In spite of her injuries, she is such an amazing person. In fact; she reminds me of Janet. If you have any further questions, please give me a call. Maybe we can go to lunch and you can tell me how it's going thus far." "That will be fine and I trust your judgment. Thanks for filling me in and I will buzz you when I am ready for lunch."

Kelly had not had a close encounter with Mr. Seward since her orientation and had forgotten how mesmerizing he was. She almost felt that accepting a lunch date would be cheating on Kevin. They had not put a label on their relationship but she had not seen anyone else since she met him. She thought that she would give him a call just to clear the air so that there wouldn't be any hard feelings. Kevin told her that he would miss having lunch with her but that he was okay with that, besides; he would be having a working lunch today with a new client.

The morning had flown by so quickly. It was 1:00 by the time that

Kelly had finished briefing her assistant and finishing up some other things that had a suspense date for today. She buzzed Mr. Seward's office to let him know that she was ready for lunch. It was raining and Kelly hated to go out in the rain. She asked Mr. Seward if the cafeteria in the building was okay. He said that it was and that he would be waiting for her in the lobby. After they had sat down to eat, Mr. Seward asked her how the temp was working out. Kelly told him that she was a charming person and that they were getting along just fine. She had never met anyone who had so much hope and joy after such a tragic event. It is so amazing how God was working in Dee Dee's life. She was a missionary in her church and often did a lot of outreach for the disabled and homeless veterans. There were days when she just did not feel like getting out of bed but often pushed herself to take care of those that have defended our nation and had been deemed as castaways by mainstream America. To her, it seemed that those that have not served, does not understand what our military men and women go through to obtain the freedoms that our nation so richly enjoy. Kelly told Mr. Seward that she would like to volunteer some of her time to help those that have served and are now a forgotten part of our society. She would bring it up in her next sorority meeting and maybe it could be one of their community service projects. Kelly and Mr. Seward continued to make small talk through the duration of their lunch. She noticed that a great number of employees patronized the employee cafeteria and it seemed that a table of ladies was starring at them. She asked Mr. Seward if he was seeing any one at that table. He said that he was happily married and was aware of the looks and rumors that floated through the office. It was flattering but he would never cheat on his wife. They were having a lot of fun these days since all of the children had moved away from home. After they had finished eating, Kelly thanked him for lunch and was glad that she had not been forward with him. He did not have a wedding band on and she thought that he was not married. She found out at lunch that he did not wear his wedding band because he had broken his finger years ago and that he had waited too long to seek medical treatment and his finger could not be reset. He wore his wedding band on a chain around his neck. He felt that as long as it was near his heart, he would always remember the vows that he had taken.

When Kelly got off work, she decided to give Janet a call to see if she had made it home. They did not talk long because Janet said that she was tired but would fill her in on everything when she got to work in the morning. Kelly told her to get some rest and she would see her tomorrow. She thought about Bennie and his in-laws but decided against calling him. She knew that he had his hands full and would talk to him some other time. Kelly thought about how it would be if something were to happen to either of her parents and decided to call them to let them know how much she loved them and missed being home with them. Did she make the right decision by being so far away? Her mom assured her that they were fine and that she needed to make a life for herself because they had lived and enjoyed a rich life. Kelly was one of their greatest joys but children are raised to leave the nest at some point. They were proud of how she had turned out and besides; South Hill just did not have anything to offer her in the way of a career. It was a settled town and people were not retiring, so career minded people had to move away if they wanted to accomplish anything. Kelly also told her mom about Dee Dee and she wondered if she would have the same spirit as Dee Dee if she had gone through something like that. It gave her a greater appreciation for the military and would like to volunteer some of her time to help them in any way possible. Kelly's mom told her that her dad wanted to speak to her for minute. Kelly talked to him for about 15 minutes before hanging up. She ran her a tub of water and just basked in the warmth and exhilerence. She was so sleepy but knew that she needed to send up some prayers for Bennie and that brave soldier that had touched her life today. She knew that after this day; she would always remember to thank a soldier and do all that she could for them to show her appreciation.

Chapter 7

Home at Last

Three weeks had passed and Bennie had not made it back yet. His mother-in-law had suffered a set back and had to stay in rehab longer than expected. Janet had gone to see him every weekend while he was away. Kelly had missed her friend Bennie so much. His replacement was okay but he was not as friendly as Bennie. She was happy when Ms. Talley informed her that Bennie would be back next week. He was waiting for his sister-in-law to come in from Germany to stay home with his father-in-law and his mother-in-law was in the capable hands of the hospital staff.

On Thursday evening, Janet called Kelly to tell her that Bennie was back and if she wanted to join them for dinner. Kelly was so ecstatic and asked what time were they going. Janet told her that it would be around 5:00 and they would be waiting downstairs when she got off. Kelly could hardly wait for the day to end. She was excited to know that she had her old driver back! Once again, Bennie had out done himself on picking out the restaurant. It was called Angie's Golden Nook. Bennie told her that Angie was an old friend from South Hill and she had just moved to New York. The establishment was decorated lavishly and served a variety of foods. Bennie said that it had only been in business for about two months. He had forgotten about it until he saw the advertisement on television last night. The friends enjoyed their meals and just sat back conversating about things that had transpired while they were away from each other. Bennie asked Kelly if her relationship with Kevin had grown into a committed relationship yet. Kelly informed him that it had not but they were spending a great deal of time together, in fact; she felt as if she was cheating on him by accepting an invitation for lunch with someone else. She was also unsure how she would take it if she were to see him with someone else. The friends continued to conversate well into the evening until Bennie said that he was mentally and physically drained and needed to get some rest. Kelly and Janet felt the same way and decided to call it a night.

The next morning when Kelly got on the elevator, she ran into Kevin. They exchanged greetings and Kevin asked her if she would be available for lunch today. She said that she would check her office calendar and give him a call around 10:00 to confirm and bid him a good day.

When Kelly reached her office, she pulled up her calendar and saw that she was in fact free for lunch. She called Kevin immediately and told him that she was free. He said that he was glad and looked forward to spending some time with her. He asked her if she would like to meet in the building cafeteria because he had a meeting right after lunch. She said that it was fine and she would meet him there at exactly noon.

When Kelly reached the cafeteria, Kevin was waiting for her at the door. She was embarrassed as she felt herself blush at the sight of him. Was she catching feelings? Kevin looked so handsome in his grey Armani suit and a crisp pink shirt. He had dimples to die for and a charming smile with fabulous white teeth. Kevin was a great catch, but was she truly ready?

Kevin asked Kelly if she would like to go out on the patio to eat. She said that she would and they proceeded through the exit door. Kelly accidentally brushed against Kevin as he held the door for her. She felt a warm feeling all over her body. Wow, what is this man doing to me, she asked herself. Once they sat down, Kevin took her hand and said the grace. She had never had that happen to her before. Was he the man that God had sent to her? They basically were making small talk and it was awkward until Kevin asked her if she was ready to take their relationship to the next level. Kelly tried not to seem too excited and told him that she was. She was nervous and could not say much else but a meekly yes. He shared with her how elated she was and that she would not regret being his lady. He said that he would like for her to fly to Atlanta with him the weekend to meet his parents. Kelly was so not expecting this! She agreed and he told her that he would call his parents to let them know that they would be arriving sometime on Saturday.

Kelly was flying high after that lunch date and could not wait to tell Janet the news. As soon as she got to her office, Kelly shut the door and leaned against it to regain her composure. After a few minutes, she said to Janet, "you will not believe what just happened to me?" "What" said Janet?" "Kevin just asked if I wanted to take our relationship the next level and wants me to fly with him to Atlanta to meet his parents!" "That is what's up girl!" I am so happy for you. I think that you deserve some happiness after your breakup with Todd. "I know. This is a dream come true but I thought that I would never be able to find someone to replace him. He was such a figure in my life. We practically grew up together and I just knew that we would spend our lives together. We shared everything but I guess that he was just not strong enough to wait for me. I kept the faith and God has truly sent me what I have been waiting for.

Where had the week gone, Kelly thought to herself? She decided to get up early to get her bags packed for the weekend. Kevin had asked her to spend the night with him because they were leaving so early Saturday morning. She agreed, with the stipulation that they sleep in separate rooms.

When Kelly got to work that morning, Bennie helped her to bring in her luggage. "Wow, how long are you planning to stay?" "It is not that much stuff," laughed Kelly. "I don't know a lot about Kevin's family or what activities he has planned for us this weekend. He wants it all to be a surprise. I hope that they will approve of me. I am just so nervous." "Kelly, you are the ideal woman for any man and I am certain that you have nothing to be concerned about. Just be yourself and you will be okay." Kelly thanked Bennie for his vote of confidence and they headed to her office. Bennie stayed a few moments longer to talk with Janet before leaving the building. After he was out of listening range, Kelly and Janet huddled in Kelly's office to talk about Kevin and the visit to his parents. Kelly shared with Janet that she was really excited and ready to be in a committed relationship. She just hoped that she was doing the right thing.

Kelly was waiting eagerly for Kevin in the lobby. He looked so debonair! "Are you ready to go, beautiful, said Kevin." "Yes I am," Kelly exclaimed. "Well then, Madam; your chariot awaits." When they reached the parking deck, Kevin told Kelly that he was going to cook dinner for her and needed to stop at the market before going to his house. The way that Kevin maneuvered in the supermarket, Kelly could tell that he was a regular shopper. She could not wait to taste the meal that he was going to prepare.

When they reached his condo, Kevin showed Kelly where she would be sleeping and told her that she was welcome to shower and change while he prepared their dinner. When Kelly got out of the shower, the house was filled with the aroma of scallop linguine and garlic bread. After slipping into lounging clothes, Kelly went to the kitchen to see if Kevin needed her help. He told her to just relax in the family room and he would call her when he was finished. Kelly reluctantly retreated to the family room to watch a movie. Kelly didn't know what to think because Kevin was such a gentleman and made her feel like a queen. Why hadn't some woman snatched him up? Kelly was glad that no one had because she would not have had the opportunity to be spending this time with him. She was certain that he was a keeper. After being engrossed in her thoughts for what appeared to be about fifteen minutes, Kelly heard Kevin tell her that dinner was ready. When she reached the kitchen, he had already pulled her chair out for her to sit down. Kevin said the grace and they settled down to eat. "This linguine is so good", said Kelly. "How did you learn to cook so well"? Kevin told her that he had grown up in a house full of women and was eager to learn how to cook. His grandmother often let him come in the kitchen with her. After they had eaten, Kevin got his shower; he asked Kelly if she wanted to watch a movie before they went to bed. Kelly said that it sounded like a great idea since she did not want to lie down so early after eating. Kevin asked Kelly to pick out a movie while he lit the fireplace and popped them some popcorn.

Kelly was not sure if she made the right choice in movies, but she was a die-hard fan of tear jerker movies and thought that T.D. Jakes,

Not Easily Broken was a good movie to see the sentimental side of Kevin. Kelly was not sure if she should be sitting so close under Kevin but he promised to be a gentleman. About an hour into the movie, Kevin received a phone call and told Kelly that he needed to take the call in his bedroom. She told him to go ahead and that she would pause the movie for him. After about 20 minutes, Kevin returned with a frown on his face. Kelly asked if he was okay and he told her that he was and not to worry about him. "I promise that everything is okay", he said. "Stop being a worry wart." Kelly smiled and resumed the movie. A few minutes later, she felt Kevin stroking her hair and moving closer to her. He must have felt her cringe and asked if he was making her uncomfortable. She said that she was just nervous because she had not been touched by a man in a while. She was then surprised when Kevin started stroking her face and told her that she was beautiful and he could feel himself falling in love with her. He gently cupped her face and began kissing her passionately. Kelly knew that she could no longer hold the emotions that had been pent in her for so many years. As Kevin continued to kiss and caress her body, she could feel the heat radiating between her legs and she began to stroke his manhood. She also allowed him to caress her womanhood and arched herself more towards him. She moaned with pleasure but decided that as good as it felt, it was not right. Kelly wanted to save herself for the man that she was going to marry. Kevin continued to confess his love for her and assured her that she was the only woman for him. After the movie was over, they decided that they should go to bed because their flight was an early one. Kevin gently kissed Kelly good night and started to his room. Kelly went to the bathroom to brush her teeth and changed into a nightgown because she hated wearing pajamas to bed. Remembering that she had not taken her medication, Kelly walked down the hall to get some water from the kitchen. When she got to the kitchen, Kevin was pouring himself a glass of wine. "I hope that I didn't startle you", he said. "No, I didn't know that you were in here. I just remembered that I needed to take my medication and came to get a bottle of water." "I am so glad that I ran into you. That electric blue gown looks amazing against your caramel color skin. You are so breathtaking and I am so happy that you agreed to meet my parents. I know that they are going to love you." He then pulled her to him and gave her a kiss. This time she did not stop him and he gently swept her up and carried her to his bedroom. He could not believe how soft she felt in his arms. As he laid her down, he pulled the straps of her gown down her shoulder to reveal her breasts. They stood so perky and firm. He cupped her breast in his hands and placed his mouth over her nipples and slowly moved down to plant kisses all over her stomach and eased his way between her thighs. Kelly had never gone this far with a man before and the pleasure was so great that she whimpered softly. Kevin asked her if she was okay and if she wanted him to stop. She said that she knew that there could never be another man for her and she wanted him to be her first and only. Kevin promised her that he would be gentle. Kevin decided that he would first use his fingers to prepare her before he entered her with his manhood. After he felt that she was ready, he gently stoked her with his manhood before fully entering her. As he entered her fully, Kelly braced herself for the pain. Kevin was well endowed and he knew that he had to take it slowly with Kelly. It felt as though they had made love for about an hour when Kelly finally rolled off Kevin and collapsed. Kevin told her that he was going to the kitchen to get something to drink and asked if she wanted anything. She told him that she would take a bottle of water. When Kevin had left the room, Kelly could not stand the way that the bed felt. She got up and noticed the blood and semen. She quickly pulled the linen off the bed and yelled to Kevin what he wanted to do with it. He told her that he would throw it in the washer and that they could sleep in the spare bedroom. He would change the linen when they returned.

It seemed that she had just closed her eyes when the alarm went off. "Is it time to get up already"? "Yes it is my love. We don't want to miss our flight, so you need to get in the shower. I will use the one in the master bath so that we will have time to grab something to eat after we check in our luggage". Kelly was so exhausted but managed to finally drag herself out of bed and walked sleepily to the shower. After she was done dressing, Kelly looked around the house for Kevin and noticed him coming through the front door. "I have already put our luggage in the car. Do you need a cup of coffee? I have a Kureg that brews single cups. Pick out a flavor and I will fix you a cup." Kelly loved mocha and decided that she could go for a cup of mocha. Kevin locked up, set the alarm and they headed to the car. Kevin opened her door for her to get in. "You are the guy that every girl dreams about and a mother prays for her daughter to have." "I did grow up with a house full of women, so I know how to treat a lady. My mom and grandmother would have killed me if I forgot how to be a gentleman or show disrespect to a woman."

Once they boarded the plane, Kelly let her seat back and placed her blanket over her. She was going to sleep all the way to Georgia. Even though the flight was only about two hours long; she was going to make the most of it. It seemed that she had only been asleep for about ten minutes when she felt Kevin gently shaking her to tell her that they were in Georgia. As they exited the plane, Kelly told Kevin that she would like to go to the restroom to freshen up. He told her to go ahead and he would retrieve their luggage from baggage claim. When Kelly returned, she noticed that Kevin and a gentleman seemed to be in a heated conversation. When he noticed her, he quickly came to where she was. "Who was that and is everything okay?" Kevin told her that it was just someone that he had known in college and they didn't always see eye to eye. Kelly decided to drop the subject and followed him outside to a waiting taxi.

Chapter 8

Meeting the Family

Kelly was amazed at the houses and their immaculate landscaping. A lot of the homes were in gated communities. Kevin told her that when he had completed college; his mother remarried. His stepfather was the owner of minor league football team and gave his mother whatever she wanted. She deserved some happiness in life and it seemed that his stepfather made her happy. She no longer had to work hard and only volunteered at the local schools as a past time. Kevin's stepfather's position afforded them the time to travel and his mother often traveled with her husband to away games. They are down to earth people and you will like them.

When the cab pulled into Kevin's parents' driveway; Kelly felt butterflies in her stomach. Even though Kevin told her that they would love her and that she had nothing to worry about; Kelly felt that they could see the sin of their lovemaking without being husband and wife. She knew that she could not pull this off with her parents. Her mom was the type that could see right through her and besides, she didn't think that her parents would give them their blessings in marriage if they knew what had happened.

When they stepped out of the taxi; Kevin's parents were waiting for them on the front porch. They had glowing smiles on their faces and ran towards them with out stretched arms. What a warm welcome Kelly thought. It sure helped to erase all of the stored up tension she had. Kevin was right; they were down to earth people. Kevin's stepfather helped Kevin to take the luggage in the house and Kevin's mom showed Kelly the room in which she would be sleeping. They were just as old fashioned as her parents and told them that they had to sleep in separate rooms since they were not married. Kelly said that she understood because her parents would not allow it in their house either. Kevin's mom told Kelly to go ahead and freshen up because they had made reservations to have breakfast at an exclusive clubhouse and needed to arrive there within the next forty-five minutes.

When they reached the clubhouse, Kelly was in awe of the scenery. Being from a small town, she had never seen a clubhouse of this magnitude before. It was lavishly decorated with Queen Anne type furniture and the windows were adorned with mauve colored drapes with white lace lining. Their food was served on the best china that Kelly had ever seen. Once they were done eating; Kevin told his parents that he had an announcement to make. Kevin reached in his blazer pocket, pulled out a small velvet box, cleared his throat and asked Kelly if she would do him the honor of being Mrs. Kevin McCall. "Oh my gosh"; Kelly exclaimed with tears in her eyes. "Do you really mean this; you want me to be your wife?" "Yes, I do", said Kevin. "We have been kicking it for a while and I want to make it official. I see how all of the guys at work look at you and I knew that I had to make a move before someone else comes along and snatches you away from me." Kevin's parents clapped in approval and they stood to give Kelly a hug and to welcome her into the family. "We are so happy for the two of you. I could not have asked for a better person to be my future daughter-in-law," said Kevin's mother. I have been waiting for this day to come. Kevin was so into his studies when he was in college, that he never brought any girls for us to meet. I guess that he was just waiting to get settled in his career and find that special someone. He has told us so much about you and that is why we were so excited to finally get the opportunity to meet you. I would like to help you and your mother with the planning stages of your wedding. I use to be a bridal coordinator years ago. I know that you are your parents' only child so I won't take over. Just tell her to call me sometime and we can discuss what she wants me to help with." Kelly told her that she would make sure to give her mother the message. "We will be going to visit them next weekend to give them the news. I don't want to tell them over the phone". Kevin's stepfather ordered a bottle of champagne to celebrate the occasion. A few of their friends came over to give well wishes to the couple.

Kevin and Kelly went with his parents to church on Sunday morning. The message that the pastor gave was befitting for the occasion. His topic was entitled, "A New Beginning". Kelly briefly thought about how she had overcome the pain and hurt that Todd had caused her and how she had to regain the trust of all men after his deception to her. She was glad that she chose to let go of the past and be able to give her heart to another man. This was truly a new beginning and she could not wait to start her new life with Kevin.

After church, Kevin's parents gave them a ride to the airport. Kevin's father helped to take the bags inside the airport and they all said their goodbyes before Kevin and Kelly went off to the departure gate. Once they were on the plane, Kelly told Kevin how she felt about the sermon and how it must have been a part of God's plan for them to attend the service today. She told him that she knew that she needed to let go of the strongholds that were keeping her in bondage. She knew that she needed to fully let go of Todd and forgive him for what he had done to her. It had been more than a year since she had seen him and thought that he had damaged her heart so bad that she would never give her heart again. She thanked him for loving her and allowing her to be able to walk into the season that God had destined for her life. She would always cherish the day that he came into her life and pledged her undying love to him forever. Kevin gently kissed her on the cheek and said that she had made him the happiest man in the world by accepting his proposal and that meeting her was also a good thing for him.

When they reached the airport, Kevin had the valet parker to retrieve his car while they went to claim their luggage. Once they were in the car, Kelly thanked Kevin for giving her such a great weekend. When they reached her house, Kevin got out to get her luggage and take them in for her. They said their goodbyes and Kevin told her that he would call her the minute that he got home.

Kelly decided that she would take her a nice long bubble bath before calling her parents to let them know that she had made it back from her trip and that she would call later in the week to let them know what time to expect her and that she was bringing someone for them to meet and wanted her to prepare a nice soul food dinner. Kelly told her mom to tell her dad hello and that she loved him before hanging up.

Bennie had the doorman to buzz Kelly on Monday morning to let her know that he was there to take her to the office. She said that she would be down shortly. She could not wait to tell her friend about the proposal. Bennie told her that he was happy for her and that she deserved someone that she was going to be faithful to her and someone that was going to make her happy. "So when are you and Janet going to take your relationship to the next level?" I love Janet a lot but now is not a good time. I wouldn't want it to cause my in-laws to have any setbacks. Even though they have met Janet and like her very much; I feel that they would think that I was trying to replace their daughter. I also would hate to put Janet in a situation that she does not need. We just plan to take things slow and if marriage is in our future; then I will embrace it with a welcome heart.

Janet was already at her desk when Kelly came in to check to see if she had any messages. She knew that she would be out of the office most of the day for a conference and wanted to tie up all loose ends before she left the office. She immediately told Janet about her weekend and the surprise proposal. Janet said that she was happy for her and would like to go out to celebrate whenever she was free. Janet asked Kelly if she had shared the news with her parents yet. Kelly told her that she had not because she wanted to tell them in person and that she would be going home for the weekend and would give them the news then.

The conference lasted until 3:00 p.m. and Kelly was exhausted. She called Janet to tell her that she would not be returning to the office this afternoon but could be reached on her cell if she got any important calls. Kelly hung up the phone and dialed Kevin's number. "Hello beautiful", Kevin said in his sexy voice. What does my girl have on her mind this hour of the day?" "I just wanted to let you know that I won't be back in the office today. I just left the conference from hell and need to take some mental time for myself. You can give me a call once you leave for the day.

Kelly felt refreshed after waking up. She decided to get a shower and call for some take out. When she got out of the shower; the doorman buzzed to tell her that Kevin was downstairs. "Go ahead and let him in." When she opened the door for Kevin; she could see that he had taken the time to bring her something to eat. "I was just going to order some take out but thanks for saving me the trip." Well, I just thought that I would have dinner with you since I didn't get to see you all day. I won't stay long because I brought some work from the office that I need to get completed." After eating their meal; Kevin and Kelly talked for about twenty minutes before Kevin told her that he needed to be getting home. Kelly thanked him for dinner and walked him to the door. Kelly cleaned up the kitchen and looked at the nightly news before settling in for the night. She said her prayers and thanked God for sending her such a great guy.

Kelly and Kevin decided to take Friday off to drive to Virginia to see Kelly's parents.

Kelly could not wait to see the look on her parents' face once they heard of her engagement. She was sure that they would welcome him into the family with grace and thankfulness for making their baby girl happy. Kevin wanted to make the announcement in church and called the church clerk to see if she could add it to the program. Kelly thought that this was a great idea. She wanted to share the news of her upcoming marriage with her church family back home.

Kelly and Kevin got on the road about 9:00 Friday morning. They wanted to wait until the rush hour traffic was over with. Kevin said that they could just take their time and cruise. They would still get to Virginia at a decent time. After they stopped to get some breakfast, Kevin hit the freeway about 9:45. Kelly reclined her seat back and settled in to get a nap. Kevin told her that he would put in a smooth jazz CD and set the cruise control. Kelly was happy about that because she didn't really get any sleep last night. She was excited about going to see her parents and telling them about her engagement.

Kelly heard Kevin call her name and she sleepily rubbed her eyes and wondered if she was dreaming but heard him say that they were in Maryland and he wanted to know if she was hungry. Traffic was heavy at the Maryland House welcome station and Kelly did not want to get lost from Kevin. They decided that they would meet each other outside of the restroom area and decide where to eat afterwards. They decided on subs since they were going out to dinner with her parents later. Kelly had a petite figure and worked hard to keep it that way. She hated eating until she was stuffed and worked out on a daily basis. That was one of the things that first attracted Kevin to her. Even though she was petite, she had a muscular build. They spent about an hour at the Maryland House eating and walking around to all of the various shops before getting back on the highway. Kelly asked Kevin if he wanted her to drive. He said that he was fine and besides, she would get her opportunity to drive on other vacations once they were married. He told her to just sit back, enjoy the ride and get her beauty rest. Besides, he said, you will need all of your rest to plan our wedding once we get back home. Kelly smiled; just thinking of being married to Kevin was one of her fondest dreams. Once she talked with her parents about the engagement; she would then set a wedding date. She wanted it to be soon because she did not want to lose the man of her dreams to another woman. Men like Kevin were hard to find.

It was about 8:00 p.m. when they finally pulled up in Kelly's parents' driveway. Kevin got out of the car and went around to the passenger's side to open the door for Kelly. He grabbed her by the hand and they walked towards the porch. Kelly embraced her parents for a moment and commenced to introduce them to Kevin. After all of the salutations were given, Kelly held her hand up to expose her engagement ring. "That is with your blessings of course", said Kevin. As long as our baby girl is happy; we will honor your request. Kelly's parents hugged her tightly and her father shook Kevin's hand and welcomed him to the family. Kelly said that she had called in advance to King's Barbeque for their reservation.

Once they got to the restaurant and were waiting for their order, Kelly spotted an old classmate sitting at a table adjacent to them. "Is that you Shelia", Kelly asked? "Yes, girl and how have you been", said Sheila. Kelly flashed her rock to let Shelia know that she had gotten engaged. "Girl, what happened to you and Todd", asked Shelia. "Todd got married while we were away at college, but I would like for you to meet my fiancé, Kevin. He is the man of my dreams. We both work for the same firm. I would like to get your address so that I can send you an invitation and maybe we can get together before the wedding. I see that the waitress has brought our food; so I will chat with you later." Kelly gave Shelia a hug and went back to her table. She told Kevin that Shelia and her were the best of friends in high school and had somehow lost track of one another.

Once they got home from the restaurant, Kevin said that he was really tired and just wanted to shower and get to bed. Kelly's mom asked her to show Kevin where the guest room was. There was a shower in the room that he would be staying in. Kelly would stay in her old room. Kelly's mom told Kevin that breakfast would be served at 8:00 a.m. and that if he wanted to sleep in; he could. She would just wait until he got up to fix him some cheese and eggs. She said that her Saturday morning breakfast always consisted of salt herrings, salmon cakes, fried potatoes, fat back, cheese and eggs and corn cakes. "I know that you are a city boy, but you will love my country cooking", said Kelly's mother. "Your daughter has told me all about country food and that is one of the reasons that I am marrying her. She doesn't cook pork for me a lot because she is so health conscious but I can't wait to taste your cooking", said Kevin.

On Saturday morning, Kelly and her mom got up early to go get their hair done. Kelly could not wait to see her old stylist and friend, Pat. She couldn't wait to tell her about her career and the love of her life. Pat was overjoyed to see Kelly and ran to embrace her before she got all the way through the door. What a joyous reunion it was! After getting their hair done, Kelly asked her mom if she felt like riding to South Park Mall just to have some girl time. Kelly's mom said that she didn't mind because she missed them hanging out on the weekends. At about 4:00 in the afternoon, Kelly and her mom were exhausted and decided to make the hour drive back to South Hill. "This was so much fun mother", said Kelly. "I miss our girl time". "Well honey, soon you will be married and your husband will be number one in your life. Your father and I have waited so long for you to get married and give us some grandbabies. That old house gets lonely sometimes and it would be nice to have grandkids to keep us busy and give us our youth back.

I regret that we only had one child, but the doctor felt that it was best. I suffered so much while I was in labor with you so much so that I was close to death. It was okay because it gave us double the love for you."

"Thanks mom. You and dad gave me the best of everything and I had a good life. I was able to go to college and you all never complained when you had to pay for me to live off campus. You and dad always worked to give me the life that some children can only dream about".

When they got to church on Sunday, the clerk congratulated Kelly and Kevin on their engagement. She asked them to stand to be recognized. Everyone applauded loudly. It had been a while since Kelly had been to her home church and was happy to see everyone. Kevin told her that he really liked the atmosphere in South Hill and that it would be a good place to come when they retired. "Wow, you do plan ahead. Yes, it is a peaceful area but I have not lived there for years and I am not sure if I would want to come back here to live. But we will see how things go. I don't think that I would like to retire in New York either, but Hopewell or Prince George might be okay."

Chapter 9

Planning a Wedding

After returning to New York, Ms. Talley and Kelly's friends decided to throw her a lavish engagement party. Ms. Talley purchased airline tickets for Kelly's parents so that they could enjoy this major milestone in their only child's life. She asked that no one mention this to Kelly so that she would be surprised. Ms. Talley also reserved the club house in their elite housing community. She also made arrangements for a band to play and her friend Vernon would play during the band's intermission. Angela's Catering promised to cater the event. Ms. Talley was excited with the way that things were falling in place and smiled in spite of herself. After speaking to some of the ladies in the office complex, someone informed Ms. Talley that she should contact Mrs. Stanislas of Jefferson Creations to do the decorating. She came highly recommended by a lot of people in the community as well.

The engagement party was held in June of 1995. It was such an emotional event that was attended by at least 200 people. Kelly was well-known by a lot of people in South Hill and her parents were pillars of their small community. Kevin was also well liked by the community in which he grew up and by his college classmates. Everybody who was anybody attended their engagement party. Money, DeeDee, Jackie and Benny were so happy for their friend. When Kelly first came to New York; she was an unhappy person but quickly settled in her new job and made friends immediately. Because of the pain that she went through because of her first love; Kelly was uneasy when it came to matters of the heart. It took her a while to warm up to the opposite sex and mostly kept all of her acquaintances strictly professional. Kevin was a confident person and gave Kelly all of the time that she needed to accept his friendship. Their friendship was genuine and eventually Kelly decided to give him a chance. To her, the relationship was a match made in heaven and to him, she was his greatest conquest.

In the weeks to follow, the happy couple finally decided on a wedding date. Kelly was a unique person and did not want a wedding in the traditional months of February, June, July or August. She loved the crisp cool colors of winter and the couple decided on a January wedding. Kelly and Kevin decided that their colors would be crimson and cream. Kelly was a Delta and Kevin was a Kappa, so they felt that the colors that they had chosen were perfect for their special day. Kevin made all of the plans and reservations for their honeymoon and Kelly and her parents made all of the wedding plans but made it a point to keep Kevin informed. Because they both came from large families; the couple decided that they would each invite 250 people. Ms. Talley took the liberty of getting the venue and entertainment for the reception since she knew New York like the back of her hand.

A few weeks after all of the wedding plans were made; Kelly felt sick. She called Ms. Talley to tell her that she would not be in on Monday and would call her later in the day to let her know how she was feeling. Ms. Talley told her not to worry and that it was probably the stress from planning for her big day. She would take care all of the loose ends of the jobs that were pressing and Janet could assist her.

Kevin called Kelly on his lunch break to see how she was feeling. She told him that she just wanted to sleep. He said okay and told her that he would stop by after work. Kevin picked up juice and soup after work and had the door man to let him in so that Kelly would not have to get up. When he got there, Kelly was asleep so he decided to let her rest. He went in the den to make a few phone calls and watch the evening news. Kelly finally woke up at 7:00 p.m. She got up to go to the bathroom and was startled when she heard the television. She peeked in the den and saw Kevin. He got up to give her a hug and asked it she wanted him to heat up some soup for her. After eating the soup and drinking some juice; Kelly sat in the den with Kevin for about thirty minutes and told him that she was going back to bed. Kevin told her that was okay and that he had brought some clothes to spend the night with her. He did not want to leave her alone in her condition.

The next morning, Kelly still was not feeling any better and Kevin made her promise to make a doctor's appointment. She assured him that she would. In the meantime, Ms. Talley called Kevin to see how Kelly was feeling. Kevin told her that she was not any better and that she would be making a doctor's appointment today. Ms. Talley told Kevin to tell Kelly not to worry about coming in the rest of the week and she would get a temp to come in.

Kelly woke up a few hours later after Kevin had gone to work. She felt so weak that she didn't think that she could make it to the bathroom alone. She needed to get up because she was shivering because of the sweating that she had done during the night. She looked around the bedroom to find something to help her steady herself in order to go to the bathroom. There was a jumbo umbrella in one corner of the room. She knew that was the closest thing to a cane. She carefully slid off the bed and held on as she retrieved the umbrella. She felt dizzy and decided to wait until the dizziness has subsided. Once she got in the bathroom, Kelly decided to call her doctor. The nurse was very understanding and told her that they had seen an unprecedented number of flu cases this season. She told her that she could come in tomorrow morning. After hanging up with the nurse; Kelly called Kevin to tell him that she had an appointment for tomorrow and if he would take her. He said it was no problem and wanted to know how she was feeling. She told him about the dizziness scare but she was okay. Kevin told her that he was going to take the rest of the afternoon off to take care of her. She told him that it was not necessary but he did not want to hear it and said that he would be there within the hour.

When Kevin arrived at Kelly's place, she was taking a bubble bath. She was hoping that if she took a bath and changed the bed linens that she would begin to start feeling better. While Kelly was in the tub, Kevin changed the bedding and sprayed Lysol through the house. He also lit some candles to make her room cozy and comfortable so that she could relax. Once Kelly was done with her bath; she asked Kevin if he could heat her some broth and crumble the crackers in it. Kelly then called her parents to tell them that she was not feeling well but had a doctor's appointment for the next day. Her mom told her to be sure to call her once she got home. She promised that she would and lay down. She told Kevin that her body was aching. He found some massaging oil in the bathroom and heated it up to rub her down. The massage was so soothing that soon Kelly drifted off to sleep. Kevin undressed and got in bed holding her while she slept. He thought how nice it would be having her as his wife but he was still confused about his sexuality. He had a past that he just could not shake. He was hoping that it would not surface once he and Kelly were married. Was it normal to have feelings for another man yet be in love with a woman?

When Kelly arrived at the doctor's office the next day; the nurse had her fill out all of the necessary paperwork while waiting for the doctor. Kevin asked her if she wanted him to accompany her in the back but she told him that she was a big girl and could handle it. When the doctor came in; he asked Kelly what brought her to his office. She explained all of the symptoms that she was having. He told her that it was probably just the flu and gave her a flu shot and prescribed a cough medicine and an antibiotic. He told her that she should stay at home the rest of the week and call if she did not get any better. "Have you been tested for the HIV virus?" "No I have not", said Kelly. "I have only had one partner and I was a virgin until recently but if you insist, then I will have one done." "A lot of people feel that they don't need one if they are in monogamous relationships but the truth is, once you are intimate with someone; you are sleeping with every person that they slept with. I have seen a number of cases like yours and sometimes they are proven to be fatal and besides; I recommend it to all of my patients. You should be safe rather than sorry." Kelly finally agreed to take the HIV test. Dr. Scranage told her that the results would be back in a couple of days and he would give her a call if the results came back positive. She said okay and walked out to the waiting area where Kevin was waiting for her. Kevin dropped off Kelly's prescriptions at the pharmacy and took Kelly home. He told her that he would go back out later to pick them up and also pick up take out for their lunch. He asked her what she wanted to eat. She told him that she was still feeling queasy and would like some wonton soup from the Chinese restaurant by her house. After dropping Kelly off at home; Kevin decided to go to the grocery store to get some tea and more soup.

While in the pharmacy, he thought about his grandmother rubbing him down in vapor rub when he had the flu or a cold. He decided that he would get some for Kelly. The florist near Kelly's house usually sold rare arrangements with stuffed animals attached. Kevin stopped there to purchase a bouquet of African violets with a teddy bear. He hoped that this would brighten her spirits.

As Kevin was entering the gate to Kelly's place; his cell phone went off. He looked at the number and it was his lover from his college days. He called to tell Kevin that he had full blown AIDS and that he should get tested as well. Kevin angrily told him that it was not any of his business and not to call his phone anymore. His friend told him that he thought he wanted to know and that he was slowly dying. He missed what they once shared and wanted to see him one final time. Kevin told him that he was getting married and this was not the time to spring some news of this sort on him. Kevin hurriedly hung up his phone and went into Kelly's building.

By the weekend; Kelly was feeling much better and went back to work the following Monday. Everyone was glad to see her and Ms. Talley had Janet to have some flowers delivered to Kelly's office. Kevin called to Kelly's office to tell her to call him if she needed anything. She assured him that she was fine and not to worry about her. After getting settled; Kelly called her mom to let her know that she was back at work and was feeling okay. She was just a little weak but that was probably from being in bed all weak. Kelly told her mom that she had to hang up because she had a lot of work to complete that the temp did not have the authorization to do. She told her mom that she loved her and promised to give her a call when she got off work.

By noon, Kelly was beat. She knew that there would be a lot of work waiting on her but did not imagine that it would be this much. Kelly decided that this would be a good time to stop and take her lunch break. She called Kevin to tell him that was going to go to the cafeteria to get some potato soup. Kevin told her that he was having a working lunch but would check on her once he was free. When Kelly returned from the cafeteria, Janet told her that Dr. Scranage had left a message for her to call him. Kelly decided to wait until after she had eaten to call him. What could he want, she thought to herself. He said that he was only going to call if the results were positive. Could he have another reason for calling her? Dr. Scranage's nurse answered Kelly's call and informed her that he wanted to see her. She asked if it could wait until she got off work. The nurse told her that she would check. When she came back on the line, the nurse told Kelly that would be fine and they would be waiting for her. Kelly did not much feel like working the rest of the day but she would have to find a way because there was so much that she needed to catch up on.

At last it was 5:00 and Kelly phoned Kevin and told him that she had an errand to run and would talk to him later. She hung up the phone and hurried to the lobby to meet Benny. She told him that she needed to go to the doctor's office and would take a taxi. "Are you sure, Kelly?" "Yes, I will be fine and tell Janet that that I will call her when I get home." Benny said okay and drove off.

When Kelly entered Dr. Scranage's office, the receptionist told her to have a seat and she would let him know that she was there. When the nurse called for Kelly to come in the back; she wondered why someone else was there. Dr. Scranage informed Kelly that he had taken the liberty to call in a psychologist due to the nature of her visit. "Why would I need a psychologist, asked Kelly?" "Please have a seat, Kelly. This is not easy but I have to tell you that you are HIV positive. I called in Dr. Jackson just in case you need someone to talk to. I have already gotten your prescriptions together and I need a list of all of your sexual partners. Kelly started to feel tears welling in her eyes and fought to hold them back. The news was so devastating that she did not know what to say. "Maybe the test is wrong or it got mixed up with someone else's test. I have only been with one guy and we have a monogamous relationship." "There is no mistake Kelly, but I will be testing you again in six months. This is not a death sentence and people have been known to live twenty years or longer if they stay on their medications and take care of themselves. You are going to need people that care about you to be there for you. If you don't want to tell your friends right away, Ms. Jackson is just a phone call away. I will also be available for you. Please feel free to call me any time." Dr. Scranage gave Kelly a hug and told her that everything was going to be okay in time. Right now she had to stay strong and not stress herself.

Kelly left out of the office in a daze. What was she going to do? How would she tell her parents and most importantly; how could she tell Kevin? They were going to be married. This had to be a dream and Kelly hoped that she would awake soon.

Kelly finally regained her composure and flagged down a taxi. Once inside the taxi; Kelly told him that she needed to stop at the pharmacy before going home. She was glad that Dr. Scranage had called in her prescription ahead of time so that she would not have to wait. She did not feel like facing anybody after her devastating news. Kelly was glad that she did not run into anyone that she knew. She did not know if she would be able to handle it. Would she break down and cry? How would she break the news to her friends and family? Would Kevin still want to marry her, but most of all; how did she get the dreaded virus?

When Kelly got home; she saw that she had four missed calls. One was from her mom, one from Janet and Kevin had called twice. She decided that she would wait until tomorrow to call her parents and Janet, but she knew that if she didn't call Kevin; she knew that he would be at her house in a flash. She sounded kind of down and Kevin asked her if everything was okay. She assured him that it was and that she was tired and wanted to get in bed early. Kevin asked her if she wanted him to come over. She told him that she would not be much company and that she would see him at work tomorrow.

By Thanksgiving, Kelly's secret was weighing down on her and she was glad to have a break from the madness at work. She called Money to see if she would be in town for Thanksgiving. Money told her that she would. "Is everything alright with you," asked Money. "Not really but we will talk when I see you."

When Kelly got to her parent's house; her mom asked her where Kevin was. "He decided that he would spend time with his family and friends since the wedding is only a few months away. Besides; I want to spend time with you guys." When Kelly opened the front door; she was hit by the aroma of collard greens, chitterlings, rolls, pies and cakes. Kelly's mom was a whiz in the kitchen and loved to cook. During Thanksgiving and Christmas; she always cooked enough to take to the battered women's shelter. Kelly went to her room to unpack her bags before going to the kitchen to help her mom out. Her dad and one of his brothers were sitting in the den watching television. Kelly's mom told Kelly that she looked like she needed to eat some of her home cooking because she was looking kinda frail. "I lost some weight when I was sick and it's been hard to eat a proper meal because I had so much to catch up on and I have been eating on the run. It won't be hard to put the weight on with your cooking this weekend."

Money called Kelly on Thanksgiving morning to see if she wanted to go out to breakfast. She told her that she was going to help her mom out at the shelter and that she was welcome to go with them. Money said that she would pass but would be over later for dinner. They talked for about another thirty minutes about the wedding and Kelly's love for Kevin.

After leaving the shelter, Kelly and her mom headed home to prepare the table for the annual feast. When they reached their driveway, Kelly spotted Kevin's car. "Kelly, I thought that you said Kevin was going to spend time with his family", her mom asked. "He said that he was, so I don't know what's going on". When Kelly walked in the door; Kevin was standing there with a bouquet of yellow roses. "Kevin, what are you doing here? I thought they you wanted to spend time with your family." I was, but you seemed down before you left and I just wanted to make sure that you were okay. I had already phoned your dad ahead of time to see if it was okay for me to come and he said that it was fine. Aren't you happy to see me?" "Yes I am", said Kelly. "I just thought that since you had not been home in a while, that you would want to see your family." "You are my family Kelly and when you are down; it is my job to keep you happy". Todd's parents were close to Kelly's parents and they usually ate with them on Thanksgiving. This year, Todd, his wife and their baby were present as well. Kelly did not mind because she was in love with Kevin and Todd was a part of her past. It no longer hurt for her to see him with someone else. They had shared some good times and felt that they would spend eternity together. His purpose in her life had run its course and she was thankful that she got to see the real Todd before it was too late. Kevin was now the man of her dreams and she was madly in love with him.

As they all sat around the table sharing their life stories and thanking God for all of their blessings; Kelly was grateful for the new chapter in her life that she was about to embark upon. When it was her turn to share what she was thankful for; she lovingly looked into Kevin's eyes and said, "I am thankful for day that I met Kevin and how our friendship evolved into a relationship that is one in a lifetime. I thank God for sending him to me. I could not have selected a better man for myself. I am also thankful for my family and friends who stuck by my side when I was going through. Life could not be better. I have a fantastic job with lots of fringe benefits, a nice home and most of all; a great man to share it all with." As she finished her speech; she could see tears welling in Kevin's eyes as he took her hand and planted a kiss on it.

After dinner was over; all of the women pitched in to clean the kitchen and the men retreated to the family room to watch football. When they had finished cleaning the kitchen; Kelly and Money went to her room to talk. "So what did you want to talk to me about"; asked Money. Before Kelly could talk; she could feel tears welling in her eyes and she just clung to Money. "What could be so wrong? You are getting married in a couple of months". Kelly felt her voice stuck in her throat as she buried her face in her pillow. Finally she gathered her composure and told Money that maybe they should talk somewhere else. Kelly told everyone that she was going to ride out with Money for a bit and catch up on girl talk.

Money told Kelly that they could go to her hotel room to talk. When they reached the hotel, Kelly was such a mess. Money was puzzled by her sadness and asked her what could have her in such a pickle. She was going to marry the man of her dreams in a few months; she had a fantastic job and lived in an exclusive neighborhood. What could possibly have her feeling like this? When Kelly was finally able to talk; she informed Money of her doctor's visit and the dreaded news that he had given her. "Aren't you going to tell Kevin what is going on"? "I don't know how. He might not want to marry me. Maybe I should just keep it to myself after the wedding. Dr. Scranage said that he would test me again in six months. Maybe it's all just a big mistake. I will tell him Money, but I just don't think that this is the right time. Suppose the first test was wrong and I would have caused problems that could have been avoided." "Okay", said Money. "I still think that you are making a big mistake. I am your friend and you have my support. You know that I am always here for you. Now get yourself together so that your man won't think that you are hiding something from him."

When Kelly and Money returned to the house; everyone was watching a movie. Kelly walked over to take a seat by Kevin and kissed him on the cheek. She was always subtle in displaying her affection for Kevin in front of her parents. She was a good kid and always tried to be respectful to her parents. Kevin was equally as glad to see her. He had sensed that something was wrong and that's why he had driven to see her. His first instinct was that Kelly has having cold feet and was having second thoughts about marrying him.

When Kelly returned to New York; she had a lot to do in order to catch up on her work before her wedding. The time seemed to just fly by and she was getting nervous and stressed with each passing day. She was about to open an important chapter in her life and wanted everything to go well. The wedding was going to take place in South Hill and she was getting stressed out trying to handle all of the arrangements from New York. Her mother was assisting her as much as possible but she didn't want her to take on all of the responsibility. She would be making the trip to Virginia in a couple of weeks for the fitting of her gown. Her wedding party would get their fittings as well. She was still waiting for the invitations to come from the printer's office. She hoped that they would come soon. She wanted to get them out in a reasonable amount of time in order to put her order in with the caterer. The wedding was the least of her worries. She still had to deal with the tragic news of her illness. Because of her positive test results; Dr. Scranage had given her medication for HIV. She had to hide it from Kevin. What was she thinking? She knew that this was not the way to start a marriage. How many lies would she have to tell to cover herself? Her only hope was that when she took another test, that it would come back negative. It had to. She had waited so long for a husband and having a family. Would she get that opportunity? How could she explain this to her parents?

Chapter 10

The Big Day at Last

Kelly and the rest of the wedding party arrived at the Bridal Boutique for their final fittings. Afterwards, they all headed to Turnin Headz for Pat to do their hair. Kevin called Kelly to let her know that he was going to pick up his tuxedo and wanted to know what time she was going to be back in South Hill. She told him that they were all going to get their nails done in Hopewell but would be back in time for the rehearsal. "Are you missing me already"; she asked. "Yes my darling. I was just checking to see if you had gotten cold feet. I don't know what I would do if you walked out of my life. I love you and want to spend the rest of my life with you." Kelly felt her heart race. Kevin always did that to her and could not imagine life without him either.

When Kevin entered the mall to pick up his tuxedo; he heard someone calling his name. When he turned around, there was stood his lover from his college years. "What are you doing here", Kevin asked. "I just wanted to give you my well wishes and maybe we can grab a bite to eat for old time sake. There is a nice restaurant in my hotel. You don't want me to tell your bride-to-be our dirty secret do you"? "Look, I will join you for lunch but that is all. After that, I want you to forget all about knowing me and the past that we once shared. I am in love with a woman now and I don't want to have anything to do with you again".

The hotel restaurant had a bar and Kevin and his lover ordered drinks while waiting for their food. After consuming about five or six shots of Tequilla on an empty stomach, Kevin let his lover convince him that he could go to his room to sleep it off. "Man, you don't need to go to your rehersal reeking of alcohol. I won't bother you". When they reached the room, Kevin passed out on the bed. After ensuring that Kevin was asleep, his lover managed to get his clothes off and lay next to Kevin. He started caressing Kevin and Kevin started to stir. He was so out of it that he did not remember that he was in the room with his lover. Kevin's lover started kissing him and Kevin was moaning with pleasure. When he finally came to; he jumped up from the bed. "What are you doing? I told you that I left that life I no longer get down like that. I am in love with Kelly and I am getting married tomorrow. Why can't you accept that? "You are a liar. You will never get over me. Kelly is just a cover up for who you really are. If you are so in love with her; then why did you agree to come to my room? You know that you wanted this as much as I did. Besides, have you told your wife-to-be your dirty little secret? Have you slept with her yet? I am sure that she will know in time and you won't be able to hide it any longer". Kevin grabbed his clothes and headed to the shower. He was so angry for putting himself in this predicament. He was hoping that the guilt of how he spent his afternoon would not show at the rehearsal. He promised himself that was done with that type of lifestyle. But was he?

By the time that Kevin reached the rehearsal, he had put the events of the day past him. He was getting married tomorrow and no one was going to come between him and Kelly. He had admired her the day that they met but she looked even more radiant today. He was sorry that he had let alcohol take over his faculties and wished that he could erase what had happened. It weighed so heavily on him that during the dinner, he asked Kelly if she had any regrets as to becoming his wife. "No I don't. Why would you even ask me something like that?" "I just wanted to hear you say that you love me and that we will always be together". She grabbed his hand and told him that he did not have to worry about her ever falling out of love with him. He was stuck with her and he better make the most of it.

When Kelly's father walked her down the aisle that day; he was so overcome with joy for his baby girl. He could not believe how fast the years had gone by and now his only daughter was getting married. He gave her a kiss on her cheek before leaving the alter to go join his wife. As Kelly's father sat through the wedding ceremony, he reflected on the life of his daughter and how much happiness she gave her mother and him. A parent could not ask for a better child. He knew from birth that she would have a bright career and any man would be proud to take her as his wife. Kelly's father was so engrossed in going over the memories of his daughter that his wife had to shake him when the ceremony was over. "Honey, we need to stand", she said. Kelly's father abruptly wiped the tears that stung his face and stood to watch the couple exit the church.

    The reception hall was extravagantly decorated by Frances of Jefferson Creations. Kelly stood in awe at the beauty of it all. There were two ice sculptures, doves hanging from the ceiling; it was truly breathtaking. The food was catered by Angela Russell; Kelly's mom's best friend from South Hill. Kelly went over to her parents and thanked them for giving her the most beautiful wedding she had eversoon.

    Kelly's matron of honor was Sherrell J and Marquitta was her maid of honor. They had been friends since high school. Her old friend Money was a bride's maid along with Janet, Dee Dee, Retha, Robbin and Stephanie. Kelly had asked Kevin to let her play brothers, Brandon and C.J. be two of his groomsmen. He agreed that if they were her friends, then he could not see why they couldn't have the honor. By the time that everyone had toasted the couple; there was not a dry eye in the room. It seemed that Kelly had impacted each person in attendance life in some way. Her parents were so very proud but also sad that they had to share their daughter with another family. They knew that they would not get to see her every holiday as they once had. They accepted the fact that they were not just losing their little girl; but was gaining a son-in-law as well. As Kelly and Kevin were about to make their exit for their honeymoon; Kelly's father asked Kevin to please take care of his little girl and if he ever felt the need to cheat on her or treat her badly, to please bring her home to them. Kevin promised him that he loved Kelly and would give her the life that any bride would want.

    After returning from their honeymoon; Kelly went to the post office to retrieve the mail that was placed on hold. There was a blank check from her parents towards the purchase of a new home. Kelly could not wait to get home to tell Kevin the news. Kevin was excited as well because it solidified the fact that he would be viewed as a straight man. He felt that he had overcome his past and he and Kelly would have a normal life together.

To celebrate their tenth anniversary, Kevin and Kelly went on a cruise to Aruba. Kelly was on cloud nine. Even as a child; she had envisioned vacationing in Aruba. She never gave a second thought that she would actually go there one day! Kevin was ready for them to start a family. They both had promising careers and could afford to do so. Kevin also wanted Kelly to ask Ms. Talley if she could find someone else to Travel for the job so that Kelly could be home more. He was having too much idle time when he got off work. He was afraid that he would start having tendencies of being with a man again. He did not want to believe the hype that he would revert back to his old ways. He wanted to believe that his past was just experimenting and that was not what he was destined to be.

When they returned from their vacation; Kelly was so exhausted and her body ached all over. She went to see the doctor after a week of feeling so bad. Her herpes outbreak was worse than it had been before. Initially, she thought that she was just irritated because of the frequency of her sexual activity while on vacation. He doctor prescribed some meds to ease her pain from the herpes outbreak and some vitamins to give her more energy. He asked her if she had discussed her condition with Kevin yet. She informed him that she had not because things were going good and they were planning on starting a family. I have researched my condition and there have been persons that have survived the odds. I am hopeful that I will claim victory in the end. I have also had a strong faith that God will heal his chosen people of illness and disease and I stand firm on his word.

It has been a year since our tenth anniversary and the chances of Kevin and Kelly becoming parents were dim. Her parents always asked if they were going to ever be grandparents. Kelly told them that they were trying but the future was looking bleak. Perhaps she was working too much and it was stressing her body. Kelly was running out of words as to why she couldn't conceive. Today was such a bad day for her. She looked at herself in the mirror and saw how her body was deteriorating.

She often layered her clothes whenever she went out but it still did not hide the fact that something was definitely wrong with her. She often went to work and straight home. Kevin felt that she was hiding something from him but dared to ask. They often argued about small things. He knew that he was the cause of what she was going through but he never let on that he knew what her symptoms were coming from. He had gone to see his doctor before the wedding. He had been in remission but was afraid that things may have gotten worse after his encounter with his lover.

Finally, the darkness of winter was over and the April rains had subsided. Kelly was happy to see the sun again and sat out on the patio with a cup of cappuccino. Kevin came out to join her. It had been so long since they had actually spent time together and had a civil conversation. Kelly was actually enjoying their conversation. He finally gave her a kiss and asked her to join him in the shower. Kelly made up an excuse as to why it was not a good idea. After he went into the house; Kelly put her face into her hands and cried uncontrollably. Why was her life such a mess? Was God hearing her prayers or was he punishing her? What had she done so wrong to deserve a punishment such as this? She knew that eventually she would get worse and her parents would have to spend their retirement years taking care of their only daughter. They did not deserve this. They should have grandchildren to boast to their friends about. What a mess I have made of my life.

When Kelly got off work that day; she was so exhausted. Just the few steps leading to the house had her short of breath. She told Kevin that she was going to get a shower and go to bed. He asked her if she wanted him to pick them up something to eat. She told him that she was not hungry and he could just get something for himself. Seeing how fragile and sick Kelly was looking; Kevin did not want to leave her home alone and decided to fix himself a salad. Around 10:00 p.m., Kevin heard Kelly coughing violently. He went to the bedroom to check on her. She looked pale in the face. He asked her if she wanted him to take her to the emergency room. Kelly shook her head yes. Seeing that she was too weak to get up; Kevin brushed her hair and put a robe and some slippers on her. He had to lift her as she was a child because she could not walk.

The doctor came in to see Kelly. He informed her that she had pneumonia. It was one of the most common symptoms of the virus. He told her that he would have the nurse to come in and start an IV. He did not know how long she would be there, but it would probably be a week or so. He also told her that she needed to let her husband know what was going on with her. She promised him that she would. It was time. She just hoped that he loved her enough to stay. The doctor asked her if she wanted a psychologist to be present when she broke the news to him. She said that she would be fine. She just needed some time to think and asked him to tell Kevin he could come in after about thirty minutes.

When Kevin walked into the room; Kelly asked Kevin to have a seat. He had a puzzled look on his face but finally faced the reality that she knew his secret. She took his hand and told him that what she needed to say was hard for her and she did not know how it had happened. She asked him to promise that he would not see her any differently than he had in the past. "You know that you can tell me everything. What is going on"? Kelly finally just spit it out. "I am HIV positive". Kevin stood up and dropped Kelly's hand. "How long have you known"; he asked. "It's been about ten years now. Can you please not tell my parents or any of our friends? I want to wait until I am out of the hospital to tell everyone the truth. Just tell Ms. Talley that I have cancer and to expect me to be out of the office for a while. I know that my parents will want to come here if they know that I am in the hospital; so just pretend that I am away for my job." "Won't they ask why you are not answering your cell phone"? "Just tell them that I am out of range for cell phone service."

Kelly was released from the hospital after a week. Her doctor told her that in order to regain her strength, she needed to take at least a month off work and come back to see him. He would then decide if she was well enough to maintain a position that would allow her to travel or come in contact with so many people.

Kevin was there to pick up Kelly when she was released. He showed no emotion but she knew that something was wrong. The ride to the house was silent and Kelly did not know what to say. She was hoping that her marriage was not in jeopardy. She reached over and rubbed

Kevin's leg. He pushed her hand away and informed her that he was leaving. "Do you blame me for my illness? You are the only man that I have ever had sexual relations with. I don't know how it happened". Kevin finally revealed the truth. "Kelly, I had a relationship with another man when I was in college. I thought that it was just two friends experimenting. I was honest with you when I said I loved you. I thought that once we were married; the feelings that I have for another man would go away. The night of our engagement party; I had a few drinks with the man that I slept with in college. I got drunk and woke up in his hotel room naked. He told me that he still wanted me and that I could never forget him. I told him that I was not that way and that I was getting married. It was already too late when we got married. I knew that I had the disease all along. I am a carrier of the disease and could possibly out live all of the persons that I have infected. I knew when you first became ill that you had contracted the disease. I was just wondering when you planned to tell me. I am going on with my life because your parents or any of our friends will not be able to forgive me. I gave notice at the firm today that I was resigning. I will be moving to Georgia. I need for you to go on with your life as well". Kelly did not know what to say. How could he have betrayed her? She loved him with every fiber of her being but now was not sure what she was feeling.

Two years after Kevin had left Kelly; her parents put her in a nursing home near them. They kept her in their home for as long as they could. They were aging and could no longer care for her because she needed to be turned every hour due to the lesions all over her body. All of her other family members shunned her and her parents. Her mom came to the hospital every day to sit with Kelly and to sing to her. Sometimes her father would come but he cried every time that he saw his baby girl in the condition that she was in. She could no longer walk and wished that God would call her home. She was ready. She felt that she had nothing else to live for.

On June 26, 2008; Kelly slipped away to glory. Her parents were at her bedside. The nurses had rushed in to try and save her, but it was too late. God had called his child home from her misery. Kelly was finally free. She knew that God would provide her a place in his kingdom.

A Mother's Tribute of Love to Her Dying Daughter

My Dearest Daughter,

As I sit here by your bed; I reflect upon the day the day that you were born

It was one of the happiest days of my life, despite all of the pain that I went through to bring you into this world; it was not in vain. You were a happy child and brought so much joy and happiness into our home. No parents could have asked for a better child.

As you lay in your crib during your early years; angels danced around you and brought smiles to your beautiful face. I would get up all times of the night to check on my baby girl. Your dad was so thrilled that he worked day and night to give us the best of everything.

When you started walking; just hearing the pitter patter of your feet was like music to our ears. You were a happy baby and brought us so much joy and happiness. We thanked God for our beautiful gift because we were told that I would never be able to bear a child.

When you were three years old; your father bought you your first pair of ballet shoes (he called them your golden slippers). You embraced ballet like it was made for you and you had oh so much grace. Whenever people came to visit; your father loved to show them what you could do. You would perform a recital of one. To him, you were a true princess. His heart is aching right now and he cannot bear to face the inevitable.

You did not deserve to go this way and I wish that I could trade places with you. Your life was much too short. I no longer feel that my life has a purpose, but I know that God is greater than my pain and will give me the strength and courage I need to go on. Perhaps my purpose is to educate other young people about this dreaded disease.

Rest in peace my baby and on some glad morning; your father and I will join you when the Lord says that it's our time. You are now God's angel and I imagine that you have golden slippers and wings that allow you to fly with grace.

I love you, but God loves you best and welcomes you into His Kingdom to look down upon us. Your purpose in this life has been served and now I must let you go.

With Love Always,
Your Dear Mother

Diary of a Dying AIDS Patient

November 9, 1995
Dear Diary:

I don't know what is going on with me. I have not been out of this bed for a week. My body is aching and I am so feverish. I've never had the flu this bad before. Maybe I should have gotten the flu shot. If I am not better tomorrow, I will try and go to the doctor.

November 10, 1995
Dear Diary:

I went to the doctor today. He gave me a flu shot and some antibiotics. I hope that I am feeling well soon. He also advised me to take an HIV test. I've only been with one person, so I agreed just so that he would leave me alone. The results should be back soon.

November 15, 1995
Dear Diary:

Today my doctor informed me that I am HIV positive! How could this be? I've only had one partner and we have a monogamous relationship. How will I explain how this happened? I'll just wait until the time is right. We will be getting married in a couple of months.

January 15, 1996
Dear Diary:

I got married today. I still have not told my husband about my situation. Things are going so good with us. I would hate to spoil the honeymoon. My parents just purchased us a $ 300,000.00 home (with my realtor's discount) as a wedding gift and we both have promising careers. He is a stock broker on Wall Street and I am a Realtor. He drives an Audi and I have a Mercedes. What more could a girl wish for?

November 25, 2005
Dear Diary:

It has been ten years now since I was diagnosed with this dreaded disease. I am free of any major symptoms except maybe a few swollen glands from time to time and my herpes outbreaks. Lucky for me, my job takes me away a lot, so he has never seen the outbreaks. My doctor says that the level of HIV in my peripheral blood has dropped to low levels but I am still infectious. Isn't it amazing how I have managed to keep my secret safe all these years?

March 8, 2006
Dear Diary:

I cannot hide my secret much longer. I have begun to lose so much weight because I cannot eat due to the sores in my throat. I am experiencing chronic diarrhea that lasts for months on end and I have developed thrush in my mouth. I am so sick and I just want to die. I have to force myself to get out of bed each day and go to work. My co workers can see that something is wrong with me but they do not question me. The doctor says that my body is failing to keep up with replacing the "T" helper cells that I have lost.

May 31, 2006
Dear Diary:

I started developing respiratory problems last night. My husband had to take me to the hospital. They said that I have pneumonia and that it is a complication of the virus. I finally had to come clean with my husband. He didn't even act as if he was surprised or upset. Maybe he loves me unconditionally and together, we can get through this tragedy.

June 6, 2006

Dear Diary:

It has been a week since my release from the hospital. My husband informed me that he is leaving me. He said that he wondered how long it would take me to discover HIS secret. You see, when he was in college; he was a down low brother. His lover passed away a few weeks before he met me. He was told that he is a carrier of the disease. His health is not as bad as mine at this point, so he doesn't want someone that is a burden to him. What am I going to do?

June 12, 2008

Dear Diary:

It has been two years since my husband left me. I have now been diagnosed with AIDS. I can no longer walk and my bodily functions have begun to deteriorate and do their own thing. I have painful lesions all over my body. My beautiful hair is now thin and I resemble a skeleton. My family and friends have given up on me and I feel so lonely. They have left me in this nursing home to await my fate but I am ready. God has been my rock and my strength. I know that he will set me free from my pain and suffering soon. I often dream of the pearly gates and the streets paved of gold. I will be surrounded by angels with billowing wings. I will have some too. Oh God please rid me soon of my plight.

June 26, 2008

Dear Diary:

Today, I am free! I guess I slipped away during the night. It's just as well. I spent these last few weeks in agonizing pain. I had no friends or family to support me except my dear mother. She is growing old and feeble but she devoted herself to me in these last days of my time on earth. She sang to me and cooled my feverish body. She prayed that God would grant me a place on high. You see, the doctors gave up on me and the nurses were too afraid to be near me. I hope that no other human will have to live this life that I have lived. I hope that someday there will be a cure, but until then; people will have to educate themselves and make good wholesome choices, so that they can live a different life than I did. My only fault was to give myself to someone that I loved and trusted and now my life is over. Thank you diary for listening to me and letting me weep on your pages.

Written by Shirl A. Jefferson

www.ingramcontent.com/pod-product-compliance
Lightning Source LLC
Chambersburg PA
CBHW020518030426
42337CB00011B/452